THE
BRAINPOWER
PLAN

THE BRAINPOWER PLAN

21 Days to Better Brain Health

Jordan K. Davis, M.D.

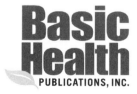

Basic Health
PUBLICATIONS, INC.

The information contained in this book is based upon the research and personal and professional experiences of the author. It is not intended as a substitute for consulting with your physician or other healthcare provider. Any attempt to diagnose and treat an illness should be done under the direction of a healthcare professional.

The publisher does not advocate the use of any particular healthcare protocol but believes the information in this book should be available to the public. The publisher and author are not responsible for any adverse effects or consequences resulting from the use of the suggestions, preparations, or procedures discussed in this book. Should the reader have any questions concerning the appropriateness of any procedures or preparation mentioned, the author and the publisher strongly suggest consulting a professional healthcare advisor.

Basic Health Publications, Inc.
28812 Top of the World Drive
Laguna Beach, CA 92651
800-575-8890

Library of Congress Cataloging-in-Publication Data
Davis, Jordan K.
    The brainpower plan : 21 days to better brain health / Jordan K. Davis.
        p. cm.
    Includes bibliographical references and index.
    ISBN-13: 978-1-59120-153-3
    ISBN-10: 1-59120-153-5
    1. Brain—Diseases—Prevention—Popular works. 2. Brain—Diseases—
Nutritional aspects—Popular works. 3. Brain—Aging—Prevention—
Popular works. 4. Self-care, Health. I. Title.

    RC386.2.D38   2005
        616.8—dc22
                                                                    2005026012

Editor: Roberta W. Waddell
Typesetting/Book design: Gary A. Rosenberg
Cover design: Mike Stromberg

Printed in the United States of America

10   9   8   7   6   5   4   3   2   1

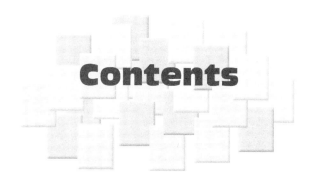

Contents

To my wife, Gale,
who encouraged me to write about brain health years ago.
I also want to honor my parents
without whose guidance I would never have gone as far as I have.
They pushed me to excel through many hardships in my life.

Acknowledgments

I am grateful to the lives of all those people who taught me the parameters by which I continue to live. In the field of neurosurgery I want to offer special recognition to the following: J. G. Galbraith, M.D., G. Harsh, M.D., S. Graham, M.D., D. Sweeney, M.D., B. Landers, M.D., and D. Brown, M.D. Their clinical judgment and surgical skills have provided an ongoing challenge for me to emulate throughout my career. They were all strong therapeutic weapons against whatever neurological condition, disease, or lesion assaulted their patients. They were true gentlemen.

I would like to thank several people who made this book possible. First, I am indebted to my wife, Gale, who has been a continuous source of encouragement, and the fire to light this project. Then to my publisher, Norman Goldfind, the editor, Roberta Waddell, and the copyeditor, Susan Andrews, for bringing this enormous work to print. Also, I want to acknowledge my son, Randall S. Davis, M.D., a physician-scientist who dedicates himself daily as a hematologist/oncologist researching leukemia and lymphoma at the University of Alabama in Birmingham. To my oldest daughter, Merrill, who is a constant source of beauty and encouragement, and to my youngest child, Jules, who knew about nutrient foods and alternative methods in high school and asked me to attend a conference on alternative health lifestyles. This was the beginning.

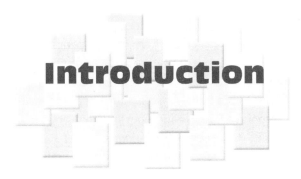

Introduction

As a neurosurgeon studying the human brain and treating its dysfunctions for more than thirty years, I know its critical importance to our health. Most people are not aware of the brain's many intricate functions, or that its high performance depends on how you conduct your life. A lifestyle that ignores the brain will promote its premature demise. As people grow older, the brain begins to decline before the body, but oxygen, a nutrient-rich diet, frequent mental stimulation, and added supplements can increase its power.

The human potential requires a new vision and a new attitude for healthy longevity. The past is riddled with myths, misinformation, and ignorance, all in the name of science, but in the past ten years, the amazing advances in evidence-based medicine have provided much useful health information. Beyond all the scientific progress, it is actually about you and the reality of self-participation and motivation, and the wise choices that protect the health of the brain—almost everything will depend on how you apply the information in this book to your life. Many people worry about dying and a life after death when they should instead be concerned about living in good health while they are alive.

Your destiny can be driven by ignorance or by knowledge. To enter a future without premature degenerative diseases, which will leave you frail and depleted, depends entirely on you. Being an active participant—a person armed with the knowledge of how to prevent such problems as smoking and epidemic obesity, two prime examples of risks for cancer, cardiovascular disease, and strokes—can only help to keep you healthy.

Today's environmental conditions are brutal for your body and brain. They can be lessened, even eradicated, by your full awareness and willingness to take positive action. Some people wish to self-destruct and there is little or nothing a physician can do about the 20 million or so depressed Americans who have willfully chosen to dismiss their responsibility for a healthy life. They do not have a vision of themselves as healthy people with healthy social interactions, which involves the need to be and think as a positive being. Caring and being cared about are vital to personal survival.

The magical brain goes both ways. It is influenced by good health and it is structured to respond to illness and poor health. Can you become ill from copious and constant data? Some psychologists think so. Information overload, while not an illness, has a negative effect on the brain and perhaps even on how people think. Too much information (TMI) has created anxiety, confusion, depression, irritability, and finally exhaustion. The bombardment of information includes negative news on TV and in newspapers, and is compounded by cell phones, e-mail, faxes, pagers, and Palm Pilots. A recent study links the onset of depression to the time spent using a computer, and another study in Britain, conducted by Dr. Glenn Wilson, psychiatrist at Kings College, London, for TNS Research and commissioned by Hewlett-Packard, found that workers who were frequently distracted by e-mails, phone calls, and text messages experienced a ten-point drop in their IQ levels. When you just can't keep up, your brain is basically malfunctioning. How do you cope with all this sensory overload? You must take the time to rest and recharge. You control the switch to all the electronic data, and *off* means you can begin to restore your brainpower.

The science journal, *Nature,* recently reported on a study from twenty worldwide institutions, which discovered that the number of human genes had been previously overstated at 100,000. The actual number has been reduced to 20,000–25,000. This is extremely important because gene identification can accelerate the diagnosis and treatment of many diseases, which can, in turn, lead to prevention, reversal, even cures. Refining the gene sequence makes the process more accurate and is responsible for the reduced number of genes. In this case, less is more. Although 15 to 20 percent of our lifespan is determined by genes, only you determine the outcome of your health.

Neuroscience has offered a new model with the discovery of brain plasticity, nerve regeneration, and replacement by stem-cell implantation. There are many facts in this book, but minimal speculation on some of the scientific studies. I do not guess about scientific outcomes, and never speculate when recommending supplements or medications.

No one should ever accept a predestined fate of neurological deficiency, illness, or the loss of brainpower. This book offers an accurate health directive to elevate your brain on several levels, including the ingestion of nutrient-rich foods, with specific supplementation to treat Alzheimer's or Parkinson's disease, and to prevent strokes. Many people may not believe they can avoid the nursing-facility experience. A healthy diet, exercise, mental stimulation, and vitamins, for example, can stave off many degenerative illnesses. Strokes, Alzheimer's, and Parkinson's disease are centered in a dysfunction of the brain, and while none of these is an absolute fate for anyone, each promotes premature aging.

I believe that aging of the brain and body is a deficiency disease, and that it is critical to take a preventive attitude concerning lifestyles, rather than attempt to treat a devastating illness *after* the battle is lost. It is out-of-date thinking to regard these diseases as natural occurrences to aging, just as cancers shouldn't be considered an expected occurrence.

This book will give you a sense of reality about your brain health. It is my purpose to make you cognizant of the risk factors for these diseases, and I will give you a plan for methods of replenishment. Informed choices can maintain and even reverse brain disease. Prevention is the new model for longevity and healthy brain function. If you are realistic and truly follow the advice in this book, you will feel and see an improvement within weeks, just as a number of my patients have.

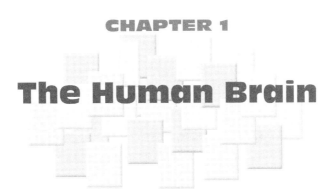

CHAPTER 1

The Human Brain

*Help! I'm being held prisoner
by my heredity and environment!*

—DENNIS ALLEN

Neuroscience is in the forefront of daily discoveries, and old myths about the brain are being debunked as it is learned that the plasticity (ability to be molded or altered) of the brain continues even into old age. Scientific evidence now suggests that by learning good health habits, you can help preserve your brain cells and boost your mental clarity. Physicians have come to believe that the risk of coronary heart disease can be altered by diet, exercise, and cessation of smoking, and by modifying other risk factors; the same applies to the brain.

The human brain contains more than one hundred billion neurons (nerve cells), which undergo apoptosis (programmed cell death) as people age. The good news, though, is that fewer cells are lost than previously thought. When I was a neurosurgical resident, I was taught that brain cells could not regenerate, but in 1998, scientists proved that the brain *does* have cells capable of dividing and becoming new healthy nerve cells, most particularly in the hippocampus, the area most crucial to learning and memory. The caveat here, however, is that in serious brain diseases, such as advanced Alzheimer's disease, cells in the hippocampus shrink and this slows down mental functioning, particularly memory and cognition.

In addition, there is a new group of diseases of the mitochondria (the engine of the cell), which reduce the number of neurotransmitters, the specialized brain chemicals required to conduct nerve impulses from one neuron to another, and this deficiency contributes to various age-related memory changes. A disruption in the vital neurotransmitter systems can make the brain malfunction and destroy memory. (Help is on the way, however—in the near future, it is expected that supplements for this, the chemical deficiency in the neurotransmitters, will be available.)

At the other extreme affecting brain function is receptor failure, meaning that the cells are not receptive to the transmitted message. As an example, in Alzheimer's disease the number of receptors for acetylcholine (a neurotransmitter involved in memory and learning) declines, as well as the acetylcholine itself, and the ability to transmit it declines, a problem that is being worked on by the drug companies. Meanwhile there are natural, nondrug steps you can take to keep your brain healthy.

Research in the field of nutritional neuroscience has demonstrated how food, supplements (including hormones), exercise, and lifestyle changes can all have an impact on brain function. Glucose and fat, in particular, can have an immediate effect on the brain regarding behavior, mood, and well-being. Dr. Richard Wurtman and his colleagues at the Massachusetts's Institute of Technology in Boston recognized that the constituents in food can be analogous to drugs in regulating neurotransmitters and behavior, which indicates that food is a regulator of brain function. And the newly discovered role of vitamins as antioxidants and neuroprotectors is no less astounding. But before any discussion of the ways in which brain disorders can be diminished in order for the brain to function at a higher level, I would like to discuss the brain's makeup.

A BRIEF SYNOPSIS OF BRAIN STRUCTURE AND FUNCTION

Neurons (nerve cells) carry messages through an electrochemical process. The brain has 100 billion neurons, all ensconced in the important cell membranes. Within the cell, the nucleus contains genetic material called chromosomes. Outside the nucleus, there is cytoplasm (jellylike substance) within the cell membrane, which contains a complex of inorganic and organic substances. The mitochondria, also located in the cell, but outside the nucleus, produce energy to fuel activities in the cell, such as cellular respiration within the cytoplasm. The neurons carry out cellular processes, such as protein synthesis and energy production. There are extensions outside the cell: multiple dendrites, which carry information to the cell body, and one axon, which takes information away from the cell body. Communication between these cells is based on a complex electrochemical process, and research has shown that, if you eat a nutrient-rich diet, take supplements, notably antioxidants, and engage in regular mental and physical activity, more of these crucial connections in the nervous system that make the brain function better can be created.

THE BRAIN PARTS

- The cerebral cortex is the outer layer (the bark) of the cerebral hemisphere— the gray matter. It covers the two hemispheres in your brain, both of which analyze sensory data and are responsible for memory, learning new information, and making decisions.

- The left hemisphere interprets and produces information on language, math, memory related to language, and reasoning.

- The right hemisphere provides a picture of your environment. Some spatial skills, such as dancing and sports, are coordinated by the right hemisphere, and auditory, spatial, and visual memory is stored there.

- The corpus callosa are white-banded fibers that connect the hemispheres for communication between them.

- The frontal lobe deals with cognitive memory; the prefrontal area is responsible for thought processes—emotions, inhibition, judgment, personality, and self-awareness.

- The motor cortex controls voluntary motor activity.

- The premotor cortex stores motor patterns and language.

- The parietal lobe processes sensory discernment of pain and body orientation.

- The occipital lobe is the primary reception area for vision and interpretation of vision.

- The temporal lobe is the receptive speech area (language comprehension), the auditory receptive area, and extends to the verbal memory and other language functions. It is also the area for retrieving information.

- The cerebellum deals with coordination, balance and equilibrium, and, to some extent, memory for reflex motor actions.

- The brain stem is the pathway for information between the brain and the body.

THE LIMBIC SYSTEM

At this juncture, the word *mind* is interchangeable with *brain* since the discussion is about the complexity of conscious mental events and what the individual feels, thinks, perceives, reasons, and expresses emotionally.

Much of the center for emotions involves structures near and in the midportion of the brain. This network, called the limbic system, plays a major role in emotional expression. The autonomic (sympathetic and parasympathetic) systems, as well as the enteric (gut) systems are part of the limbic nervous system. It is the sympathetic and parasympathetic pathways that constrict or dilate the blood vessels and that can enhance or diminish the emotional process.

The limbic system, known as the primitive, or old, brain has direct connections with virtually all parts of the brain and spinal cord, and together these constitute the central nervous system. It plays a major role in memory and processing, as well as in expressing emotion. The system is also responsible for instructive behavior and motivation. The expression of anger, fear, joy, and sadness, and the workings of the digestive system are due to changes in the limbic system. The major portion of this system is composed of the following:

- **The amygdala.** All your varied experiences in life, your negative and positive emotions, are encoded here for the brain to provide personality and memory.

- **The cingulate gyrus.** This connector between the limbic system and the cerebral cortex regulates social behavior.

- **The hippocampus.** This is located inside each temporal lobe. It has a major role in learning, memory, and what you experience personally. In declarative memory (memories that can be verbalized), factual material is preserved within the hippocampus. The hippocampus transfers information from short-term memory to long-term memory.

- **The hypothalamus.** This unit regulates critical activities: appetite, hormonal levels, temperature, and sexual activity. Its connection with the pituitary gland and endocrine system means that it plays a vital role in the composition of spinal fluid and blood.

- **The thalamus.** This is the main relay center for sensory impulses to the cerebral cortex. It also acts as the receiver for all the senses except smell. The thalamus and amygdala work to encode new memories, while storing emotions at the same time.

When the limbic system in the brain is not stimulated, people can become lifeless and dull—if they ignore their emotions and thoughts, they may stop feeling. Over time, these ignored inner feelings become so painful that the brain severs the neural connections between awareness, which resides in the limbic system, and other parts of the limbic system, which causes the person to lose touch with emotions and reality. The limbic system is involved in anger turned inward, which can result in depression, a mental state that is epidemic today. More people in this country are being treated for depression now than ever before in history, which explains the rage for antidepressants.

When anger is directed outward, it can result in cruelty, violence, and adamant denial. The callousness and insensitivity people can show today has desensitized everyone to the point of turning off and not showing emotion. The result is apathy, followed by anger and a diminished sensitivity of the self.

The husband and wife team, Rubin and Raquel Gue, have experimented with the orbital frontal cortex area that is involved in the modulation of aggression, and the amygdala area of the brain that is responsible for vexation and anger. The balance of these two parts of the brain is important. When this orbital frontal cortex area is damaged, a person is unable to keep his or her temper under control.

After comparing magnetic resonance (MRI) studies of the prefrontal and frontal area of the cerebral cortex, scientists found that women have a significantly higher volume of frontal cortex than men. The size of the amygdala remains the same, which suggests that when anger is aroused, women are better equipped to moderate it than men.

In evaluating relative intelligence, researchers at the University of Pennsylvania state that, although men have larger heads than women, that does not make them smarter. Women have a higher processing capacity.

There is a correlation between anger and aggression when lesions affect the frontal lobes, and it has been found that the anger expressed by people who have strokes is related to the site of injury. A study published in the *Journal of Neurology* described the inability to control anger and depression as a symptom of brain injury rather than a result of depression in people with strokes.

Teenage anger and aggression have been studied and there is evidence that the prefrontal cortex (part of the limbic system) may not be fully developed until age twenty or twenty-one. This means that parents need to put the lid on their children's anger until their young brains mature.

The most popular theory regarding the emotional connection is researcher

Candace Pert's theory of molecules and emotion. This theory involves pep-tides (amino acids) that allow emotions to originate in both the head and the body. She states that every move, function, or thought is influenced by emo-tions because emotions are peptides that bring messages to all the body's cells. She suggests that people's emotions are molecules and exist in concrete bio-logical form, a theory that explains why and how health is affected by emo-tions. If these peptides are indeed people's emotions, then they are enmeshed in everyone's systems, including the nervous system—and the emotional state (anger, joy, sadness) is related to different peptides being released and sent throughout the body. Good feelings may release endorphins (made of pro-teins with analgesic properties natural to the brain) into the communication pathway. If this theory is scientifically valid, then each peptide would experi-ence its own emotional mood.

Connections to the cortex from the limbic system allow your emotions to reach conscious awareness. Most animals rely on instinct for survival, but humans are able to rely on what has been learned and remembered, because the human brain is more developed than an animal brain. The left side of the cerebrum controls the ability to use language as the communication tool and to solve problems using logic. The right cerebral hemisphere controls most of your feelings and creativity.

THE PRIMARY FUNCTION OF THE BRAIN—COGNITION

There does not need to be an inevitable mental decline as people age. Age-related cognitive decline usually begins at fifty, but new studies have shown that the regeneration of neurons is a reality, beginning deep in the brain and migrating to the cerebral cortex, the seat of higher cognitive decline. This means it is important to take a probrain-regeneration attitude toward revers-ing brain damage in order to preserve its good-to-excellent function through-out life by providing the proper nutrients to nurture these cells. For optimum functioning, cell membranes require fortification with supplementation, and keeping elevated cholesterol at bay is extremely important so it does not impede cerebral blood flow.

Methods of Maintaining Good Cognitive Functioning

A study published in *The Journal of the American Medical Association* (*JAMA*), November 13, 2002, and sponsored by the National Institutes of Health (NIH) shows that training sessions of two hours a week for five weeks improved memory, concentration, and cognitive abilities in adults sixty-five years or older. The methods used helped older people maintain good-to-excellent cognitive status as they aged, and could be applied to tasks they do every day, such as handling finances or taking their own medications.

Another study at the University of Illinois at Urbana-Champaign, demonstrated that some key areas of the brain, which are adversely affected by aging, could be modified by fitness. Aerobic exercises boost the cellular and molecular components of the brain. Exercise improved problem-solving and other cognitive abilities in older people. A high-resolution MRI demonstrated the anatomical differences in gray and white matter between the physically fit and the less-fit aging patients. The areas of difference were in the frontal, parietal, and temporal regions.

Researchers at New York University studied people with diabetes in relation to cognitive function. It is known that the supply of glucose to the brain is reduced in diabetes, and that the impaired metabolism of glucose is associated with cognitive decline and memory impairment. The hippocampus is particularly vulnerable to an inadequate sugar supply, and this can eventually cause atrophy.

Neuroscientists at UCLA have demonstrated that personality and cognitive capacity are most likely hereditary. A 2001 study published in *Nature Neuroscience* suggested that intellectual ability, as measured by intelligence tests, corresponded closely to the genes of the subject's parents.

As neurologist Paul Thompson said, "We were stunned to see that the amount of gray matter in frontal brain regions was strongly inherited and also predicted an individual's cognitive test scores—the brain's language areas were also similar in family members. Brain readings that were found to be most similar may be especially vulnerable to diseases that run in families, including some forms of psychosis and dementia."

The loss of libido in older people is caused by a depletion and/or hormonal dysfunction of the adrenals, testosterone, or thyroid. This loss can lead to depression, but it can be successfully treated by supplementation, once it is diagnosed.

The pinkish-gray brain, composed of fat and water and weighing about three pounds, is amazing and requires care. The brain does not increase much in size after the age of three, and it develops most of its potential for learning during these first three years of life, a critical time when creation of the communication pathways for the brain cells begins.

The Shrinking Brain and Cognitive Function

C. Edward Coffey, M.D., chairman of Henry Ford Health System's Department of Psychology in Detroit, Michigan, said, "Our research shows that education does not reduce brain changes associated with disease or aging, but rather enables more educated individuals to resist the influence of deteriorating brain structure by maintaining better cognition and behavioral function."

In essence, the study found that people with a higher level of education exhibit more severe brain shrinkage with age than people with fewer years of education. This research involved 320 healthy men and women, ages sixty to ninety, living independently in the community. They were screened for impairment using a mental status examination. An MRI measured the size of their brains by seeing whether or not there was an increase in cerebrospinal fluid around the outside of the brain, and the results showed that brain shrinkage, as evidenced by more cerebrospinal fluid outside the brain, was significantly greater in people with a higher education. Despite the greater brain shrinkage, however, the bottom line is that both the men and women with the higher education demonstrated no severe impairment of memory or the thinking process, which showed that education was effective in buffering their brains against memory loss.

Memory and Cognitive Function

Memory is a process of recalling what has been learned and retained. Memory failure is complicated. It is often related to energy failure, which can be secondary to a faltering transport system for the cell's insulin-glucose level or to the mitochondrial power plant within the cell not getting enough of an energy boost to activate its processes. What is crucial to memory is not the *number* of cells, but the brain's ability to effectively conduct the electrochemical reactions between the neurons—this is the critical factor for cognition, intelligence, memory, and mood. If there is mental decline, the reasons can include depression, low vitamin-B_{12} levels, ministrokes, side effects of medication, stress, thyroid disease, and others.

Dr. John Rowe at Mount Sinai Medical Center in New York said it right: "People are largely responsible for their own old age." (And I would include their brainpower in this quote.)

Most of the research related to memory and cognition function is produced by drug companies in conjunction with sometimes-slanted university drug trials. The market for brain boosters, or cognitive enhancers, is huge, and growing, as the aging population grows. Excluding Alzheimer's disease, the goal of this vast market is to provide drugs (even with their potential for harmful side effects), or (safer) supplements, which can prevent the memory deficits that even healthy older people experience. Memory loss or dementia can also be caused by multiple sclerosis, Parkinson's disease, or schizophrenia. Many of the newer compounds seek to improve the way recent memory is stored and transferred into long-term memory.

Keys to Healthy Cognitive Functions

- **Emotional balance.** This includes a sense of purpose and meaning. Social and family contacts, spiritual convictions, and a sense of humor all lead to a more pleasant and balanced individual. Also, having financial stability has an enormous affect on emotional stability.

- **Mental activity.** Critical thinking and education promote plasticity (flexibility) and the enhancement of electrochemical connections between neurons. People with college degrees are less vulnerable to memory loss or dementia than those with less education.

Cognitive Functioning Slides Downhill

Jason is a sixty-year-old retired dentist whose cognitive function began to dwindle over a two-year period, slowly affecting his quality of life. MRIs of his brain revealed multiple white-matter lesions, which are visualized as small, bright patches below the cortex. Although white-matter lesions are viewed as a normal part of aging found in those with no hint of a dementia or neuro-cognitive disorders, they are closely linked to such health problems as hypertension and other risk factors. Since Jason had not taken his hypertensive drugs as often as directed, his blood pressure vacillated. He was actually undertreated, leading to brain lesions, which contributed to his cognitive decline. The additional blood tests revealed a marked deficiency of magnesium and zinc. Supplementing these minerals has renewed Jason's interest in his hobbies, and in addition, his energy has increased.

- **Physical activity.** Hundreds of research articles stress that the brain requires oxygen, which it cannot store. Regular exercise enhances circulatory health, which promotes adequate oxygen delivery. Exercise helps develop new brain cells in regions as important as the hippocampus.

I have written this book as an advocate for your brain's health. In each of the following chapters, I emphasize the many paths to prevent your brain from aging. Much of the data comes from the best available evidence and the conscientious use of it when it comes to making decisions about the care of individual people. That is what the practice of evidence-based medicine involves—integrating a physician's clinical expertise with the best available research.

Advances in neuroscientific approaches spanning the last five to ten years have improved brain health. If you follow the advice in this book and focus on supplements, exercise, mental stimulation, and moderate lifestyle changes, you will see improvement within three weeks, just twenty-one days, as many of my patients have.

CHAPTER 2

Diseases of the Brain— Strokes

I might repeat to myself, slowly and soothingly,
a list of quotations beautiful from minds profound—
if I can remember any of the damn things.

—Dorothy Parker

Age is a physiological process not necessarily connected to physical age. Medically speaking, biological age and chronological age are separate, which is to say that two fifty-year-old men can be years apart in their physiological makeup.

Later chapters will discuss how your biological age can advance for the better, but first I need to focus on the three primary diseases of the brain. In this chapter, I will concentrate on strokes (brain attacks)—the third most common cause of death after heart disease and cancer, and the most preventable of all. This is followed by Alzheimer's disease and Parkinson's disease in the next two chapters.

Sadly, most of the traditional medical establishment continues to view these conditions as the unavoidable consequences of aging. In fact, genetics (the medical equivalent of fate) plays a significant role in only 15–20 percent of the population.

No one is immune to chronic disease. If you are serious and use preventive measures, however, you can escape these diseases. If you have a stroke, Alzheimer's, or Parkinson's, you can keep the perils of impairment and disability at bay. Consider the information and act on it.

A plethora of proven research data, from stem cells to gene modulation, shows that longevity medicine's boast that everyone has an opportunity to live 120 years or more is, in fact, an attainable goal. However, if you are ill and incoherent, having a long life without your health is nothing more than a punishment.

The goal here is to avoid that by improving the quality of daily life, which, I fervently believe, can be achieved through diet, lifestyle, supplements, and other aspects of a personalized regimen that promote brain health. These measures will reduce the terrible disabilities that can occur with the three primary diseases of the brain, and their effects can be felt within twenty-one days.

Risk factors hold the key as to who will have strokes or who will end up with Alzheimer's or Parkinson's disease. Your commitment to making the necessary changes to improve your health, and perhaps the health of those you love, can lead to better health and lower the chances of these risk factors. You can be the messenger for prevention.

STROKES—BRAIN ATTACKS

Although strokes (brain attacks) can be extremely debilitating, many people are oblivious to the threat. Even those who are aware of the statistics are more than likely uninformed about how to prevent strokes or lessen the severity of the damage they cause.

Every year 750,000 Americans have a new or recurrent stroke. And 160,000 people die from their first stroke. The level of disability, requiring extreme financial resources as well as caregivers' energy, is insurmountable. The American Stroke Association (ASA) wrote that, in 1999, strokes accounted for one of every 14.3 deaths in the United States, costing the nation nearly $50 billion in direct and indirect costs.

In February 2002, an ASA survey of 1,000 people indicated that one person in ten said that strokes were the health threat they feared most—35 percent of the respondents said someone close to them had experienced a stroke. Yet few people recognize the symptoms of a stroke. Although, from watching television, even young children know the symptoms of a heart attack like clutching the chest and losing consciousness, few have seen anyone on TV having a stroke. Hippocrates, considered the father of medicine, called a sudden cerebral event *apoplexy* (the word for suddenness in his language). If you had sudden, severe chest pain, plus pain down the arm, you would suspect a heart attack and call 911. On the other hand, though, if similar events affect the brain, you might do nothing—even physicians sometimes do nothing.

Causes and Symptoms of Strokes

Both the heart and the brain require a constant supply of blood, which carries oxygen and nutrients to them (25 percent of the body's oxygen is received by the brain). When the blood is not flowing, a heart attack or a brain attack occurs, caused either by a blockage or a rupture of a vessel, which disrupts the normal blood flow. A disruption in the flow of blood to the brain is the primary reason for a stroke.

The symptoms of a stroke can be less dramatic than those of a heart attack—dizziness, loss of balance, slurring of speech, or diminished vision—or they can be as severe as complete paralysis. The severity of the impairment depends on how long blood flow to the brain was disrupted.

A sudden or rapid onset of any of the following symptoms can indicate a stroke and should be treated immediately. If you or anyone you are with experiences any of these, immediately call 911 and go to the nearest emergency room:

- Dizziness
- Loss of sensation in an extremity
- Partial loss of vision
- Slurred speech
- Sudden falling
- Unexplained loss of consciousness
- Unsteadiness

Types of Strokes

There are several kinds of brain attacks, each requiring different treatment and prevention measures. If you experience any of the above symptoms, first get medical attention immediately. You can learn later what type of stroke it was.

Transient Ischemic Attacks (TIA)

Ischemia means a deficiency of oxygen in vital tissues. Should any of the above symptoms, particularly blackout, dizziness, and weakness, appear suddenly and then go away just as fast, this could be a transient ischemic attack, or a ministroke. This happens after blood flow has been temporarily disrupted. A

TIA is a serious warning since you are now ten times more likely to have a full stroke.

Ischemic Strokes

An ischemic stroke includes strokes caused by a thrombus (blood clot) or an embolism. Blood flow is impeded due to a blocked blood vessel. Ischemic strokes are the most common type, accounting for more than 80 percent of all strokes.

- **Thrombotic strokes.** These blood-clot strokes account for 60 percent of all ischemic strokes. The clot forms as a result of arteriosclerosis (hardening of the arteries), when the blood vessel continues to narrow in spite of an attempt by the immune system to heal it. This narrowed area in the artery, vulnerable to injury, prompts an inflammatory response, which creates a buildup of cells, in turn creating more narrowing (stenosis) and causing the blood flow to slow down. This continues until the blood vessel is completely obstructed, which paves the way for a thrombotic stroke.

- **Embolism.** This is a clot that arises from an organ or blood vessel and travels to a blood vessel in the brain, causing an obstruction of flow and the death of tissue (infarction). The heart is the most common point of origin for an embolism, as for example in people with atrial fibrillation or valvular disease.

- **Hemorrhagic strokes.** The symptoms of a hemorrhagic stroke are an altered mental state, a headache, nausea, seizure, or vomiting. A subarachnoid hemorrhage (SAH) is the result of a ruptured aneurysm (ballooning and weakening of an arterial wall), which bleeds into the brain. This condition may occur genetically in certain families. The symptoms of a brain

Two Types of Brain Hemorrhages

An intracerebral hemorrhage involves destruction of the brain tissue caused by leakage of blood into the brain substance. A subarachnoid hemorrhage occurs when an aneurysm ruptures and blood remains within the subarachnoid space, as opposed to blood within the brain tissue. Either can be combined with the other, increasing the risk for tragedy. The symptoms and signs can be the same for both.

hemorrhage are similar for both an intracerebral and a subarachnoid hemorrhage. They are:

- Confusion
- Loss of consciousness, total or partial
- Nausea and vomiting
- Painful, stiff neck
- Sensitivity to light
- Sudden, severe headache (the worst ever)

Controllable Risk Factors for Strokes

There are a number of risk factors for strokes that you *can* control.

Alcohol

Alcohol is a double-edged sword for most people. A recent study reported in *Stroke* found that light and even moderate drinking appeared to protect older men and women from developing silent strokes, small blockages in the brain's blood vessels. On the other hand, too much alcohol caused atrophy or shrinkage of the brain, due to the damage it caused within brain cells.

Diabetes

The vast complications of diabetes are strong risk factors for strokes, and are especially prominent risk factors for an ischemic brain attack. Seven percent of the men and women who die of strokes have preexisting diabetes. Strokes occur two to four times more frequently in those with diabetes than in those without it, and the long-term outcome for the first group is far less favorable than for those without the disease. Compared with other risk factors, such as hypertension, lack of exercise, and obesity, people with type II diabetes are much more apt to have a stroke. Hypertension occurs in 40 percent of those with diabetes, and it is a major risk factor for the progression of atheroma (plaque).

Elevated Cholesterol (Lipid Levels)

Lowering cholesterol may not be enough to prevent a stroke. There are ways to bring the LDL (bad cholesterol) down, but it is more difficult to boost the HDL (good cholesterol) because HDL is not diet-related. However, exercise, the cessation of smoking, and weight loss will raise the HDL.

Elevated Homocysteine Levels

Homocysteine is an amino acid, a building block of protein that is produced in the human body. At high levels, it can irritate the blood-vessel lining and cause obstruction and arteriosclerosis; it can also cause cholesterol to change into oxidized low-density lipoprotein (LDL), which is damaging to the arteries. If your homocysteine level is high, you may not have enough of the B vitamins B_6, B_{12}, and folic acid, so supplementing with these lowers the homocysteine level. Although laboratory values differ, it is my recommendation that your homocysteine should not be higher than eight. A diet of fruits and leafy green vegetables is ideal for achieving this. When supplementing with B_6, B_{12}, and folic acid, it is necessary to recheck the homocysteine level in six to eight weeks to note a positive effect.

Homocysteine and its relationship to vascular disease were discovered twenty-five years ago by Kilmer McCully, M.D., then a Harvard pathologist. Despite early resistance to his findings, subsequent investigations linked homocysteine to 15 percent of heart attacks. And a recent article in *The New England Journal of Medicine* reports that it raises the likelihood for significant carotid artery obstruction. In the March 2003 issue of *Stroke*, a report indicated that the total homocysteine level is directly related to the risk of ischemic stroke. Another 2002 study in *Stroke* found that participants with elevated homocysteine levels are more likely to suffer a spontaneous carotid artery dissection (damage to the inner lining). These account for 20 percent of all ischemic strokes, and are characterized by a sudden, severe pain in the neck. This study is the first to link a genetic angle to the complex relationship between the homocysteine gene and this type of stroke.

Obesity

Obesity may increase the risk of ischemic and hemorrhagic stroke, independent of other risk factors. Metabolic syndrome is a term referring to five negative factors that can be controlled: abdominal obesity, an increase in triglycerides, hypertension, insulin resistance (insulin resistance is the inability of the body to respond to and use the insulin it produces), and low HDL (good cholesterol). If you have the five negative factors in this group, your risk for a heart attack (myocardial infarction) and stroke is more than double. (*See* Chapter 11.)

At the 52nd Annual Scientific Session of the American College of Cardiology in Chicago, Illinois, from March 30 to April 2, 2003, data from 1988 to 1994 were collected, and they reaffirmed what I have discussed here about the traditional risk factors for myocardial infarction and stroke. To be treated for metabolic syndrome, you should avail yourself of a consistently better diet and exercise program. It's not magic, and it has proven to be successful.

Smoking

Smoking causes one out of six strokes. Anyone smoking a pack of cigarettes a day has two and a half times as much risk for stroke as a nonsmoker. Smoking becomes even more lethal when the smoker is hypertensive, and the risk doubles with each added factor, such as diabetes. About five years after you quit smoking, your risk of stroke will be cut in half. It takes five years or more to reach a nonsmoker's level of risk.

According to an article in *Circulation,* smoking is a risk factor for ischemic stroke and subarachnoid hemorrhage from a ruptured vessel. A recent study by Dr. Tobias Kurth of Brigham Women's Hospital in Boston provides further evidence that smoking is a risk factor for hemorrhagic stroke. Another study in Italy, carried out by Professor Gallo of Perugia University, involved 416 people. Half of these people had had strokes and more than 40 percent of these strokes had occurred in the heavy smokers.

Even if you do not smoke, but live with someone who does, their second-hand smoke will increase your risk of a stroke by 30 to 80 percent.

Uncontrollable Risk Factors for Strokes

There are many risk factors for strokes that you *cannot* control.

Age

The risk of stroke increases with age. The chances of experiencing a stroke double every decade after age fifty-five.

Gender

Although men are at a higher risk for strokes than women, strokes are clearly not just a man's disease. An interesting study from the University of Texas School of Public Health, Houston, showed that 28 percent of women reported nontraditional symptoms of strokes, as opposed to 19 percent of the men. Traditional symptoms, such as imbalance and hemiparesis (weakness or partial paralysis on one side of the body), were reported more often by men than women. Women experienced more neurological symptoms than men, including face pain (even chest pain), gait abnormality (ataxia), headaches, pain in a limb, palpitations, sensory loss, shortness of breath, and weakness of comprehension, focus, and speech. These symptoms were not only less traditional, but less specific, and for acute strokes an accurate diagnosis is critical for successful treatment.

Heredity

Close relatives, such as a parent or a sibling who has experienced a stroke, will garner a greater risk for you. The impact of each specific gene as it relates to an individual has not yet been determined, but a number of genes associated with heart disease and hypertension, as well as strokes, have been reported. There is a tendency for fatty deposits in arteries and heart disease to develop over many generations, and a family history of hypertension, heart disease, or stroke will increase the near-certainty of strokes in close relatives.

At the University of Texas, Dr. Eric Bowin studied a gene for strokes by tapping into more advanced knowledge of the genetics of hypertension, the main risk factor for stroke. This gene (GNB_3) demonstrated that it increased strokes in Caucasians by 1,523 times, but did not affect the risk in African Americans. His research showed that this gene acts apart from hypertension and therefore is an independent risk factor for strokes. In the near future, genetic research may lead to preventive treatment.

Race

African Americans have a greater risk of brain attacks than other population groups, and those who live in the southern United States have the highest mortality rates from strokes. As recorded in the *Atlas of Stroke Mortality,* the Centers for Disease Control and Prevention (CDC) conducted a seven-year study with West Virginia University and the University of South Florida, and the data collected from 1991 to 1998 showed that 40 percent more African Americans were likely to die of strokes than were whites.

The CDC has confirmed a ten-year trend of racial disparity in the increased incidence of cancer, heart disease, and strokes for African Americans. The fatality rate due to strokes was 166 out of 100,000 for blacks, the rate for white adults over the age of thirty-five was 1.4 times lower. Almost half of all stroke deaths among African Americans occurred before the age of seventy-five, compared to 25 percent for whites.

The CDC held that poverty and socioeconomic factors explain the racial and geographic disparities, but it is my belief that common sense, as well as diet and exercise, certainly play a part. (Many of those studied were obese as well.) The highest rates of strokes are in the coastal plains of the Carolinas and the Mississippi Delta, and the lowest are in New Jersey, New York, and Massachusetts. Because of this disparity, the clear need for more education in nutritional matters to prevent strokes is being addressed nationally.

The Prevention of Strokes

To prevent or lessen the severity of strokes and the damage they cause, it is important to know as much as you can about the causes. The analogy to cardiovascular disease is clear, since most heart attacks happen after a blocked blood vessel causes an infarction (death of tissue). The brain vessels are similar to those in the heart and are affected by most of the same biomarkers (an indicator of an event to come). The good news is that most strokes are preventable, if the risk factors and symptoms are recognized and treated before the event.

The Importance of Nitric Oxide

Nitric oxide is an important component of stroke prevention. The inner lining of the blood vessel is a delicate tissue called the endothelium. The discovery that nitric oxide is produced in the endothelium was considered so important that in 1998 the Nobel Prize in Medicine was awarded to the American researchers who made it. This oxide is a molecule that keeps the blood vessels healthy and protected. However, most Americans are not producing enough nitric oxide in their blood vessels, mainly due to the prevalence of such risk factors as elevated cholesterol, hypertension, obesity, smoking, sugar, and aging itself, which all act to decrease its production. Each of these risk factors damages the endothelium of the vessel, which reduces the production of nitric oxide, and consequently weakens a person's self-defense against heart attacks and strokes. On a positive note, however, the endothelium has the capacity to repair itself and produce more nitric oxide when these risk factors are replaced with a healthy regimen.

Nitric oxide has many functions in the body. It can:

1. Open blood vessels, keeping them relaxed and pliable to increase blood flow.

2. Prevent arteriosclerosis by not allowing platelets (clotting particles) and white blood cells to stick to the walls of the blood vessels.

3. Reduce premature aging by reducing the production of free radicals.

4. Suppress the growth of vascular muscle cells. Blood vessel walls consist of layers of smooth muscle cells and elastin for contraction and relaxation of their walls. When there is an injury or inflammation affecting a blood vessel, the muscle cells become active, divide, and migrate into the hollow vessel. This activity can cause an obstruction in the vessel similar to hardening of the arteries.

If blood vessels are not healthy, they constrict and their walls eventually thicken. The blood cells can then congregate inside these walls, creating blood clots or arteriosclerotic plaque. If the endothelium in blood vessels *is* healthy, it releases nitric oxide, which relaxes the blood vessels and prevents cells from sticking to the vessel walls.

Protecting and Repairing the Endothelium

Keeping your endothelium healthy requires a low-fat diet, a frequent exercise program, and supplements designed to stimulate the body's natural mechanisms to fight vascular disease. Treatments for protection, regeneration, and repair of the endothelium are:

1. Antioxidants: flavonoids and carotenoids

2. B vitamins

3. Exercise

4. L-arginine and phytoestrogens, especially daidzein and genistein

5. A modified Mediterranean diet (emphasizing a variety of beans, cereals, fruits, nuts, seeds, vegetables, and whole grains)

6. Omega-3 fatty acids

7. Salt reduction if you are hypertensive (this will lower your blood pressure and have a positive effect on your endothelium)

ADMA and Strokes

ADMA, asymmetric dimethylarginine, is a modified amino acid, which can block the production of nitric oxide. In an important discovery, Dr. Salvadorre Moncada and Dr. Patrick Vallance of the Glaxo Inc. Research Institute/Wellcome Research Laboratories in Kent, England, found that patients with known kidney failure had accelerated hardening of the arteries and were at high risk for strokes and heart attacks because they had high levels of ADMA.

They discovered that higher levels of the arginine-like ADMA molecules in the blood vessels worsens the vessel disease by blocking the beneficial effect of L-arginine itself, thereby causing a decreased production of nitric oxide. This is significant for people who experience peripheral arterial disease.

Japanese scientists used ultrasound on the carotid arteries of 120 subjects in a study and found a similar effect in their brain arteries. Those individuals with an increase in ADMA had thicker blood vessels in their brains and more plaque. This group of scientists in Tokyo also proved that a higher elevation of ADMA in the blood is an independent marker for vessel thickening in the brains of women, indicating that carotid arteries and arteries in the brain are similar in men and women.

Dr. John Cooke and his group at Stanford University summarized the results of the relationship of known risk factors to stroke and heart disease, as well as their relationship to ADMA levels, by stating: "ADMA is a common pathway through which all risk factors exert their adverse effects on the blood vessel wall. ADMA accumulates in people with risk factors and ADMA blocks the production of nitrous oxide, causing poor blood flow and contributing to hardening of the arteries." ADMA elevation indicates an increased risk for endothelial dysfunction and future negative vascular events.

Antidepressants and Strokes

The combined use of serotonin-enhancing antidepressants—the serotonin-reuptake inhibitors (SSRIs), Paxil, Prozac, Wellbutrin, and Zoloft, for example—with migraine drugs that also enhance serotonin (triptans such as Imitrex and Zomig) may increase the risk of a stroke because too much serotonin can restrict blood flow to the brain. Since the antidepressants increase the level of serotonin in the blood, the risk of combining them with the migraine drugs is very real—there are 28 million people with migraines, and 20 million of these have depression. If you use this combination of drugs and have symptoms of a sudden, severe speech problem, you should consult your healthcare practitioner.

Aspirin and Strokes

A study presented at the February 2000 Meeting of the American Stroke Association in Phoenix suggested that baby aspirin (81 mg) or coated aspirin might not be as protective as previously thought. This study of more than 250 people showed that those who took low-dose aspirin had no reduction in blood clotting, and that a full-size, *uncoated* aspirin seemed more effective, based on platelet functions. About half of those who had heart attacks or strokes were taking low-dose aspirin (81 mg) at the time.

The director of the stroke program at Northwestern Memorial Hospital in Chicago found that 56 percent of the people taking 81 mg of aspirin had no changes in blood clotting, but 72 percent of those taking 325 mg of aspirin had measurable effects. This study also showed that coated aspirin produced a lesser reduction, or no reduction at all, in clotting. In April 2002, the journal *Circulation* mentioned aspirin resistance in those people who may be resistant to its antiplatelet action. ASA (aspirin) should help protect a person from a cardiovascular or cerebrovascular event, such as a heart or brain attack. To measure effective ASA for such an event is critical. The resistance may be the ability of the ASA to produce an effect on your clotting mechanism, such as platelet function, inhibition of thrombaxane (a clotting factor), or the lack of inhibition of platelet aggregation, also necessary for clotting. Studies reveal that many people taking low-dose ASA (about 50 percent) have a heart or brain attack. All of this information further emphasizes the need for you to know the effectiveness of ASA. Studies have found ASA resistance in up to 30 percent of ASA users. It is best to ask your physician to check whether aspirin is working for you.

The Verify Now Aspirin Test is simple and measures your platelet aggregation. The numbered result indicates whether ASA is effectively inhibiting platelet function, or if you are ASA resistant. The results of this test are available in thirty minutes, and the cost of the test is covered by Medicare and by most insurance providers. Again, testing the efficacy of the aspirin being used may be very important.

Bacteria and Strokes

The ulcer-causing bacteria, *Helicobacter pylori*, have been shown to increase the risk of heart disease by causing inflammation of the arteries. In addition, new research from Rome indicates that this bacteria can produce a toxin that damages the endothelium (the lining of the blood vessel), thus promoting a clot that can cause strokes. Treatment for the infection of *Helicobacter pylori* can help prevent such strokes.

Diet Pills and Strokes

The use of diet pills is now associated with ischemic strokes. As reported in the January 2002 issue of *The Journal of Neurology*, diet pills may trigger strokes, so you need to be aware of the drug combinations you are taking. And according to researchers at Yale University, people who take over-the-counter (OTC) diet pills have a greater risk of strokes. They found that weight-loss preparations, such as Dexatrim and AcuTrim, can increase the likelihood of a hemorrhagic stroke by sixteenfold. Phenylpropanolamine (PPA), an OTC stimulant for the central nervous system, has been responsible for more than thirty deaths since 1979, and although the manufacturers refute the scientific evidence, in November 2000, the FDA announced a ban on the sale of PPA in products without a prescription.

Ephedra and Strokes

Not all herbal medicine is benign. Ephedra is said to aid in weight loss, but the isolated concentrated components sold for this purpose can produce seizures, palpitations, and abnormal heart rhythms, as well as psychotic reactions. In a study at the University of Michigan, the rate of hemorrhagic stroke tripled in those using high doses of these concentrated isolates of ephedra. They have been removed from the general market, and their use for athletic performance, muscle building, or weight loss, is prohibited.

Note: In their haste to react to the alarming reports, the regulators acted on only a fraction of the story. The real story is that ephedra is one of the best bronchodilators on the planet and the Chinese have used the whole plant, with its built-in protective balancing qualities, for centuries without harmful effects. It was only when manufacturers started isolating the ephedrine in it and boosting it to dangerously high levels that the trouble began. In nature, ephedrine accounts for only 1 percent of the plant's substances, about .5 mg in the whole plant. Contrast this with the *20 mg* of ephedrine in *each* manufactured herbal drug pill. Of course this was bound to cause problems, but the problems are with the isolated herbal drug ephedrine, not with the whole plant ephedra itself. This crucial difference was ignored, and as a result, an extremely valuable whole plant is no longer available in this country for the natural relief of allergy or asthma conditions.

Estrogen and Strokes

In 2002, the medical profession was caught unawares by a study from the Women's Health Initiative, which found that the combination of estrogen plus progesterone as hormone replacement therapy for postmenopausal women had serious drawbacks.

The study, based on the synthetic drug Prempro, not on natural bioidentical hormones, found that HRT (hormonal replacement therapy) was associated with an earlier risk of stroke (the year before, an increased risk of breast cancer in postmenopausal women on HRT had already cast a bad light on this regimen). The risk of strokes with combination therapy was elevated during all five years of the study. It had previously been thought that this combination therapy was protective; however, the statistics for the study are impressive. There was a 41 percent increase in strokes and a 27 percent increase in heart attacks with the combined therapy. The rate for blood clots in the legs and lungs doubled. The complementary approach is to switch to bioidentical hormone therapy, which does not have the side effects of the synthetic regimen (based on smaller studies).

Fish and Strokes

A twelve-year study conducted at the Harvard School of Public Health and reported in *The Journal of the American Medical Association* (*JAMA*) on December 25, 2002, revealed that 44,000 men who ate fish once a month or more reduced their risk of ischemic stroke by 44 percent. I strongly recommend eating fish once a week or more.

Flu Infections and Strokes

A flu infection can destabilize a plaque deposit in a major artery, triggering the formation of clots in the blood supply to the brain and heart. A February 2002 study in the journal *Stroke* highlighted the role of infection in causing strokes, and reported that those who took flu shots had fewer strokes. If there are no contraindications, you might consider having an annual flu shot.

Periodontal (Gum) Disease and Strokes

Periodontal disease is an independent risk factor for stroke, particularly ischemic stroke. Inflammation in the vessel wall plays an essential role in the progression of arteriosclerosis and the erosion and rupture from the plaque.

Neurologist, Mitchell Alkand, M.D., of Columbia University in New York, stated, ". . . periodontal disease may not just be a problem with oral hygiene in the loss of teeth. It may, in fact, present a problem with cardiovascular health, neurological function, or loss of life as well."

Research presented at the American Association of Neurology meeting in April 1999 indicated that periodontal disease was a risk factor for thickened carotid arteries, which can lead to strokes—they found that the people with the worst periodontal disease had the thickest carotid arteries. The risk of heart attacks and strokes is two times greater in people with periodontal disease, so it is strongly suggested that periodontal disease should be treated aggressively and that concerned dentists should refer people to their physicians for stroke and heart-attack evaluation. Anyone who has had a stroke needs a careful oral-cavity exam to prevent a recurrent stroke.

In connection with this, C-reactive protein (CRP) is a sensitive marker for inflammation, and there is a simple blood test for this. The inflammatory reaction caused by an ischemic stroke is measurable by the CRP concentrations, which are said to predict the outcome of strokes. Periodontal disease and elevated CRP levels could be useful markers in identifying anyone at high risk for strokes. Daily dental hygiene and the use of anti-inflammatory supplements can reduce the incidence of strokes. This book utilizes the latest scientific information regarding inflammation, which has proven to be either a cause or an effect of disease, and is today's health buzzword.

According to numerous studies, CRP is a better indicator for the risk of heart and brain attack than the standard cholesterol test. CRP is a measure of inflammation in the arterial walls, and is a prime risk factor itself. You may not be aware that close to 50 percent of those who experience a heart attack have *normal* cholesterol levels, so there is a need to devise tests and treatment to reduce this risk. Do not be lulled into complacency by low cholesterol—get your CRP level tested.

Potassium and Strokes

An eight-year study in Hawaii, which monitored 5,600 men and women over the age of sixty-five, indicated that people with low-potassium intake in their diets are one and half times more likely to have strokes, and found that those taking diuretic drugs for hypertension had very low potassium levels. Potassium sources include avocados, bananas, citrus fruits, green leafy vegetables, milk, and nuts.

Statins and Strokes

A stroke is a risk following a heart attack, so lowering cholesterol is a factor in reducing risk for stroke after a heart attack. Investigators at the University of California reported that lowering cholesterol levels helped prevent strokes in people who had suffered heart attacks. A group of 3,086 test subjects were divided—some were placed on cholesterol-lowering drugs (statins), while others received placebos. The group on the statins suffered fewer strokes than those on the placebos. This is an ongoing study so we should be hearing more about it in the future.

However, good medicine insists that prior to taking a prescription for statins, a person must make a commitment to reduce his or her elevated cholesterol, triglycerides, or LDL (bad) cholesterol. Diet, exercise, and the reduction of total fat intake (saturated and unsaturated) and, of course, sugar should be the goal. This is doable for most people who are serious about avoiding heart and brain attacks.

For those who cannot reduce their cholesterol through diet and exercise, the current drugs of choice are the statins. More than 24 million people use statin drugs in this country now. A statin is a coenzyme A (HMG-COA) reductase inhibitor, which works by blocking the enzyme in the liver responsible for the production of cholesterol. Side effects with these drugs are common, despite the rhetoric of the drug companies. Common side effects include:

- Abdominal pain
- Constipation
- Decreased sexual performance
- Diarrhea
- Dizziness
- Flatulence
- Headaches
- Heartburn
- Insomnia
- Skin rash

Less well-known side effects include:
- Blood-pressure fluctuation
- Blood-sugar vacillation
- Muscle symptoms including tenderness, weakness, and a condition where the muscles undergo destruction
- A negative effect on liver function
- Ringing in the ears (tinnitus)
- Swelling in the joints
- Vision changes

All of these side effects are serious, and some can be fatal. In addition, you need to know the following:
- Antifungal drugs can interact negatively with statins.
- Depression, mood changes, and even psychosis and suicide can occur (there are 25 million Americans who are clinically depressed), and people whose

depression was caused by statins show an improvement when they discontinue the drugs.

- Grapefruit juice has an absolute effect on liver metabolism. A chemical in this juice turns off a liver enzyme involved in metabolizing statin drugs. This can cause high blood levels of the medicine, increasing the risk of muscle damage (a known side effect). Therefore, when you are drinking grapefruit juice, do not ingest statins.

- Infections and antibiotics can interact with statins, causing damage to your nervous and muscular systems.

- Memory and concentration can be negatively effected. Some people report "holes" in their memory. Cognitive function is reduced while taking statins.

- Pain in the form of headaches or joint discomfort are common.

- Peripheral neuropathy—burning, numbness, or tingling sensation—may be dose related, which will often improve when the statin drug is discontinued.

Finally, a very important fact unexposed by the drug makers is that there is a reduction of CoQ_{10} levels in people taking statins, and supplementation is mandatory. The neurological complaints related specifically to the brain can be secondary to inadequate levels of CoQ_{10} (*see* Chapter 7 for additional information).

Many physicians are not familiar with the scientific evidence on problems related to the side effects of statins. Such concerns as insomnia, irritability (mood changes), and memory deficits are truly off the radar for many of them. The motivation to use natural remedies can often prevail, if only to avoid the need for another prescription.

Stress and Strokes

As reported in the March 2003 issue of *Stroke,* a Danish study followed a large group of men and women for thirteen years and found that those individuals who reported a high level of stress were twice as likely to have fatal strokes as those with less stressful lives. The problem with this study, however, is that the highly stressed participants were more likely to engage in unhealthy activities, such as drinking or smoking, that could lead to hypertension, and less likely to engage in regular physical exercise that could lower hypertension. Reducing the associated risk factors for stress, and therefore the stress, might show that the stress by itself was not the culprit.

Vaccines and Strokes

The National Institute of Neurological Disorders and Strokes have been test-ing a vaccine that reduces chronic internal inflammation. The tests on labo-ratory animals have shown that far fewer strokes have occurred in animals receiving the vaccine than in the control animals that did not get the vaccine. The study, reported in the September 2002 issue of *Stroke,* is the beginning of an attempt to produce a vaccine that reduces internal inflammation.

Weather and Strokes

A study conducted in Dijon, France, revealed that specific weather conditions had an influence on the type of strokes people have. For example, higher air pressure and humidity are risk factors for blockage of the larger blood vessels, and temperature affects circulation. There is ongoing research on the subject, which may reveal how to cope with weather conditions to reduce the risk of strokes.

Awareness Is Critical

Any delay in recognizing stroke symptoms delays obtaining crucial treatment. In case anticoagulation, clot busters, or surgery are indicated, they are all on a tight timeline to prevent or limit disability. A stroke must be recognized as a medical emergency. The May 2002 issue of *The British Medical Journal* had an article entitled, "People Don't Recognize Stroke Symptoms," emphasizing that common symptoms—weakness of one side of the body, blurred vision, slurred speech, difficulty swallowing, dizziness, and confusion—may occur and need to be recognized as stroke threats. Stroke education needs to target those who are at risk.

A 2001 study reported that more than 30 percent of those who experienced a transient ischemic attack (TIA) and called their primary care physicians were neither evaluated nor sent to hospitals within the necessary window of time following the first event. This indicates that even medical professionals dis-miss the symptoms of stroke and the importance of early treatment.

Diagnostic Tools

A duplex ultrasound scan is a simple, safe, and painless test that uses sound waves to generate a picture of the artery (usually the carotid) and the blood flow through it. The test is interpreted by the percentage of narrowing and the degree of blockage.

A computerized tomography (CAT) scan is a computerized x-ray of the brain. It gives images that can determine whether a stroke actually occurred. High-speed CAT scanning improves the accuracy and detail—it can distinguish between an ischemic and a hemorrhagic stroke. (The former is caused by a clot in the blood vessel and the latter by a burst of blood from the vessel.) The location of the damage needs to be pinpointed accurately. Utilizing a helical CAT scan requires injecting contrast dye into a vein in the arm, which then allows the technician to view the blood flow inside the vessels and record the pattern of blood distribution throughout the brain.

A magnetic resonance imaging (MRI) scan produces detailed pictures of body tissues and organs without exposure to radiation. The electromagnetic energy exposes a patient to radio waves in a magnetic field and is measured and analyzed by a computer. The images can be two or three dimensional and are projected onto a monitor.

A magnetic resonance angiogram (MRA) scan is an MRI study of blood vessels. A special form of contrast dye may be injected through a vein to make the MR images crisper. This painless procedure is very useful in diagnosing blood-vessel problems in the carotid arteries and in the brain.

Treatments for Strokes

Surgery

An accurate diagnosis of an aneurysm (a ruptured vessel) or a blood clot requiring evacuation is the only reason for surgery. A 2003 report in *Stroke* discusses the inappropriateness of surgery for blocked arteries in some people. The number of endarterectomy operative procedures to clear blocked arteries in the neck has dropped in volume since the 1980s, but one in ten people still have the procedure done, even though the risks may outweigh the benefits. Carotid endarterectomy is beneficial for those who have at least a 60 percent plaque occlusion of the artery, but researchers found that 27 percent of the people who had this surgery did not have sufficient obstruction of the arteries to warrant it. Quality radiological studies can accurately determine the amount of blockage.

According to Professor Ethan A. Hall, M.D., at the Mount Sinai School of Medicine in New York, more attention needs to be focused on evaluating a person's overall illness before they have the surgery, especially when blockage without symptoms is found.

The recommendation is that people who are symptomatic, with temporary strokelike symptoms, are required to have at least a 50 percent blockage before they consider having an operative procedure. And asymptomatic people should have at least a 60 percent blockage before they consider having the procedure. And they should seek a second opinion.

Surgical Procedures

A carotid angioplasty or endarterectomy removes obstructing plaque. Another procedure, an extracranial-intracranial bypass, which may be helpful for some but has had mixed results, involves taking a healthy artery in the scalp and rerouting it to an area of the brain that is deprived of blood because of a blocked artery.

Recovering from Strokes

Appropriate monitoring and aggressive treatment is required when a person is recovering from a stroke. The risk factors that led to the stroke must be reduced at the same time that medication is prescribed, and a review performed. A program of anticoagulation for an ischemic stroke should be considered, and the person's care should be managed by a stroke specialist. If you have any concern that you might have risk factors for a stroke, you should seek out a hospital that has a stroke unit and team before any tragic event occurs.

In addition to neurological damage, people with strokes are at risk for blood clots, deep-vein thrombosis, pneumonia, pulmonary embolisms, urinary tract infections, and other serious problems that can reduce survival.

Poststroke Therapies

More than 90 percent of those who survive strokes experience some degree of improvement following rehabilitation, but unfortunately, some cost-cutting regimens may not allow appropriate rehabilitation. In a logical or rational world, specific rehabilitation should be determined by the deficit resulting from the stroke, not by the amount of money that can be allotted to the rehabilitation.

There are effective therapies available to restore nerve cells after a stroke, and they include antioxidants, particularly carotenoids, which help preserve the integrity of brain tissue so that less cellular damage results.

Emergency Measures for Strokes

Initial Steps in Managing a Brain Attack

Do not waste time calling the family doctor. Call 911 instead. This emergent crisis is time-sensitive. Time will dictate whether or not you survive and will also determine how much disability you experience. Going to the hospital in an ambulance shortens the delay in getting treatment. Receiving treatment early is critical to reducing the damage from a stroke, and anyone arriving at the emergency room by ambulance, versus those who arrive on their own, always gets immediate attention.

Upon admission to the hospital, an emergency CAT scan is necessary to determine whether the stroke is ischemic or from a hemorrhage, because this dictates the treatment. While in the hospital, you should receive basic support to reduce agitation, stress, and any pain that might occur. Electrolyte balance, a chemical balance of calcium, potassium, and sodium, is essential. And if your blood pressure is elevated, it must be treated promptly.

Information and Action

A Canadian study in *The Journal of the American Medical Association* (*JAMA*) in September 2002 revealed that, although strokes are the third leading cause of death in Canada, stroke prevention and therapeutic measures are not always initiated. Some important treatments are often either overlooked or not known by the physicians. For instance, anticoagulation therapy is known to reduce the risk of strokes in anyone with atrial fibrillation (a type of irregular heartbeat), yet few over the age of seventy-five are receiving such treatment.

Cell transplantation is sometimes an effective treatment for strokes. As reported in the August 2002 issue of *The Journal of Neurology,* in animal studies, bone-marrow cell transplants have improved function after strokes when the bone-marrow cells migrate to the damaged areas of the brain and produce growth factors, which help to repair brain tissue. Research on this continues.

In June 2005, a stroke treatment team in Seoul, Korea, performed a direct injection of stem cells into brain tissue that had been damaged as the result of a stroke. They reported definite improvement in the person's status and no cellular rejection.

A person who survives a stroke is at risk for osteoporosis and bone fractures. Some studies have shown that the risk for hip fractures is four times greater in people who have had a stroke. There is a tendency for fractures to

Lifesaving Unit

People with acute strokes admitted to a stroke-care hospital unit can literally have their lives saved by being in this unit. It reduces the length of their hospital stay and also reduces the chance that the person will require subsequent care in a nursing home facility.

occur on the more immobilized part of the body, usually during a fall. When a poststroke fracture happens, it is likely to be fatal, and preventive antiosteoporotic measures should be taken.

Therapies to restore and protect nerve cells following a stroke should also be considered. With the goal of limiting neural damage, paramedics in most large cities can administer treatment to stroke patients within an hour of the onset of symptoms. Magnesium sulfate (MG) is a neural-protective drug that dilates blood vessels and can prevent the buildup of calcium in brain cells, which is detrimental to cell function. A research study at the University of California, Los Angeles, conducted in cooperation with paramedics, determined that when magnesium sulfate is given within an hour of the onset of symptoms, the brain is protected. The results of this expanded, ongoing trial will probably indicate lower mortality and disability following a stroke.

Awaiting FDA approval are several neuroprotective drugs that may stop the cascading process of nerve-cell destruction following a stroke. These agents are targeting the excitatory amino acids, such as glycine and glutamate, to neutralize their destructive process.

The American Academy of Neurology suggests that giving aspirin within forty-eight hours of an acute stroke can reduce death and disability rates, as it does in heart attacks. Uncoated aspirin stops platelet cells from aggregating and forming clots. The type of stroke must be diagnosed, since aspirin would be counterproductive, even dangerous, with a hemorrhage into the brain that would contradict any form of anticoagulation.

Linoleic acid, which is found in vegetable oils, can reduce the chances of an initial or secondary stroke and has been shown to improve brain circulation. It also lowers hypertension. The sources for this protective substance are notably corn oil, soybeans, and sunflower oil.

A new antiplatelet agent, Abciximab, improves the outcome of an ischemic stroke, even when administered six hours after the onset of symptoms, and The *British Medical Journal* reported that ramipril, which is an angiotensin-converting enzyme (ACE) inhibitor used to treat hypertension, may benefit people at a high risk for strokes. A study of 9,000 people for more than four and a half years revealed that ramipril reduced the frequency of strokes in people thought to be at high risk by 32 percent, and fewer of them had physical or mental impairment than did those who did not take ramipril. The researchers suggested ramipril for people considered high risk whether or not they had high blood pressure or took other medications.

Hyperbaric Oxygen for Treatment for Strokes

Dormant brain cells that have ceased to function following a stroke may be stimulated by pure oxygen administered under atmospheric pressure in a hyperbaric chamber. By breathing pure O_2 at 1.5 times the normal atmospheric pressure, more O_2 is dissolved into the blood plasma and other body fluids, and the impaired cells may be saved. The combination of hyperbaric O_2 therapy with clot-busting drugs may be the best early-on treatment available for nonhemorrhagic stroke.

Poststroke Diet

Do you know that a fast-food meal negatively affects your blood vessels for hours? Just one high-fat meal will cause deterioration in the endothelium (blood-vessel lining), and its function will be impaired for several hours after ingesting such a meal.

Dr. Robert Vogel at the State University of New York (SUNY) studied blood vessels with ultrasound to observe the relaxation of an artery in the arm. He checked a group of young, healthy people with no risk factors for arteriosclerosis before and after they ate fast-food meals. Two hours after the meals, these participants had measurable increases in blood-fat levels, and the endothelial function had deteriorated to 50 percent of normal in all of them. The good news is, Dr. Vogel's research revealed that these adverse effects could be lessened or prevented by eating foods high in antioxidants.

By continuing to eat unhealthy high-fat meals on a regular basis, you are placing plaque in your vessels and causing an increase in arteriosclerosis. This will cause long-term damage to your blood vessels and promote brain damage. A good diet, on the other hand, improves blood flow and rewards you with healthy blood vessels and less risk for a catastrophic event, such as a heart attack or a stroke. So, take a bag lunch to work. Be creative and prepare your own balanced, nutrient-rich foods.

Calorie Reduction = Longevity

The right diet is essential to good blood-vessel health, and it has been known for many years that calorie restriction increases longevity in test animals, as well as in humans. Choosing smaller portions of food at each meal you eat daily is crucial and requires consistency and self-discipline.

A 2003 study published in *The Proceedings of the National Academy of Sciences* indicated that mice fed every other day were protected from diabetes and Alzheimer's disease. Dr. Mark P. Mattson of the National Institute on Aging in Baltimore said, "The mice are better off on a diet where they eat fewer meals . . . than when they have continuous access to food." This was more effective than just reducing calories. Although the research was done on another species, Dr. Mattson said the findings suggest that for healthy humans, often foregoing a meal "may be beneficial."

Maintaining a healthy weight means controlling the portion size and the calorie content of the food you eat; it also means using self-control. Think small portions. Read the labels and note the portion size of one serving—the size of a deck of cards represents a good portion. A nutrient-rich diet plus moderate exercise will keep you and your vessels (endothelium) in good shape.

There are thousands of diet books and diet plans available, but it is my opinion that the Mediterranean-style diet is best to protect your blood vessels—the people of Crete, for example, boast of their longevity and lack of cardiovascular disease and stroke. There is a consensus among health professionals that the Mediterranean diet is healthier than American or Northern European diets because it contains more fruits, vegetables, grains, nuts, and olive oil. The Mediterranean diet is really a lifestyle diet, as it consists of the locally grown fresh foods of the region that the people have consumed for centuries.

Research over the past thirty years has suggested that olive oil, a monounsaturated fat that is a key part of the Mediterranean diet, may actually increase HDL (good) cholesterol. Comparing the Mediterranean lifestyle to the American lifestyle, few dairy products are consumed; red meat is used sparingly; fish consumption is high; wine is consumed in moderation almost daily; and the people of this region incorporate physical activity into their daily lives, which helps maintain their optimal weight.

In a 1994 issue of *The Lancet,* a discussion of the Mediterranean diet suggests replacing butter and cream with canola oil and olive oil for salads and other food preparations. Frequent use of these oils with omega-3 fatty acids protects the blood vessels. The no-stroke diet emphasizes whole foods, such as unbleached, unprocessed wholegrain breads (never white bread); fruits and vegetables; and beans, cereals, legumes, nuts, and seeds.

I do not recommend boycotting fat altogether, as some fats are beneficial and they are needed for cells to function and for the storage of hormones. These beneficial fats carry important fat-soluble vitamins, such as vitamins A and E. You can get 30 percent of your calories from fat, but be careful about the type of fat you ingest. It is important, for example, to stay away from saturated fats. They cause blood vessels to stiffen, and blood flow requires flexibility of the cell membrane, which can be accomplished with mono- or polyunsaturated fat.

To obtain the maximum blood-lipid protection from oxidation, you should focus on foods high in antioxidants, L-arginine (nuts, legumes, and soy products), and omega-3 fatty acids. L-arginine and proteins balanced with healthy fats will provide this protection.

Free Radicals

Free radicals are unstable molecules (the smallest particles of atoms), and because they are unpaired, they attempt to gain stability by stealing electrons from other molecules, such as protein, fat, and DNA. There is little discrimination on the part of these free radicals, which destroy enzyme systems and kill cells. The toxic chemicals produced by these disruptors kill more cells and create a vulnerability to diseases, producing a very negative impact on our health. Free radicals play a major role in cerebrovascular damage. When oxygen levels are reduced, as occurs in ischemic (blood-flow reduction) brain tissue, oxygen becomes a contributor to free-radical damage.

Researchers have been unable to measure the numbers of free radicals directly; however, they have noted the processes, such as lipid peroxidation (enzyme breakdown–oxidation process), protein oxidation, and DNA damage, that mirror the production of free radicals. Every single unpaired electron looks for a mate. This process damages structure and DNA. It is a major cause for inflammation, cancer, heart disease, Alzheimer's, and Parkinson's disease, as well as premature aging.

Neuroprotectants

This group of medicines and natural products protect the brain from secondary injury caused by brain attacks. Among them are calcium antagonists, glutamate antagonists, opiate antagonists, special antioxidants, apoptosis (programmed cell death) inhibitors, and citicoline.

Cannabinoids

Cannabinoids are potent protective antioxidants in people who had strokes or head injuries. This group of antioxidants fights free radicals and helps to balance an excessive glutamate release resulting from an insult to the brain. Research indicates they may slow the progression of neurodegenerative disorders.

Carotenoids

Carotenoids are potent antioxidants that may slow the development of arteriosclerosis by inhibiting the oxidation of low-density lipoproteins. As an additional antioxidant function, carotenoids (15 mg) may help protect the integrity of brain tissue by scavenging free-radical oxygen molecules that cause cellular damage.

Citicoline

Citicoline is a phosphatide normally found in cells. If oral citicoline is taken in the first twenty-four hours after a stroke, it increases the probability of a complete stroke recovery within three months. Studies with more than 11,000 subjects have shown that treatment may reduce infarction (death of tissue). It also limits the severity of the stroke and reduces disability or death rates.

Coenzyme Q_{10}

Coenzyme Q_{10} (CoQ_{10}) is an antioxidant that helps vitamins C and E reduplicate themselves and reduces the oxidation of cholesterol in blood-vessel walls. It is important to note that the statin medications (including Lipitor, Mevacor, Pravachol, and Zocor) taken to lower cholesterol have the negative effect of reducing CoQ_{10} levels in the body. I recommend supplementing with 30–100 mg daily.

Fish Oil

Fish oil supplementation includes omega-3 fatty acids, which reduce high triglyceride levels. Coldwater fish, such as herring, mackerel, and salmon, are good sources. Omega-3 improves endothelial health, reduces triglycerides, and is an anti-inflammatory for the endothelium. If the oil supplement has a fishy odor or taste, it may have undergone oxidation and may be rancid. Avoid it because oxidation of fish oil generates free radicals. Since many fish live in polluted water contaminated by heavy metals, there is now a process of manufacturing EPA and DHA from algae because the algae are free from such contamination. Take 1–2 grams of fish oil per day.

Flavonoids

Flavonoids are isoflavones that destroy free radicals and limit the oxidation of LDL (bad) cholesterol. Soy phytoestrogens are also called isoflavones and are anti-inflammatories as well as antioxidants. Genistein, daidzein, and glycitein are major isoflavonoids found in soybeans. Isoflavones help to conserve calcium and lower blood cholesterol. Recommended dosage is 300 mg daily.

Garlic

Garlic reduces cholesterol, lowers blood pressure, and produces mild anti-platelet activity by increasing the activity of nitrous oxide.

Ginkgo Biloba

Ginkgo biloba is an herbal extract that has been used with some success in peripheral arterial disease, secondary to a decrease in circulation of the extremities. Studies have shown an increase in cerebral circulation as a result of taking ginkgo. Recommended dosage is 160–320 mg daily.

Caution: If you are taking coumadin, warfarin, or aspirin, be aware that ginkgo biloba can affect blood clotting, so you may have to avoid it.

Ginseng

Chinese ginseng has been used in China for centuries to treat disease and aging. Its effect on mild-to-moderate dementia after a stroke was not reported until recently when documented animal studies showed that Chinese ginseng caused an increase in the activity of the brain's acetylcholine. At the 28th American Stroke Association Conference, a paper reported that ginseng might help improve memory in people with a mild dementia following a stroke. Further studies are ongoing. Recommended dosage is 200 mg, two to three times per week.

L-Arginine

L-arginine, an amino acid that restores the production of nitrous oxide (NO) and can improve blood flow, requires high doses because it is utilized to make several substances including the neurotransmitter agmatine. Higher doses are also needed to overcome the elevation of ADMA, which was previously discussed regarding its interference with the production of NO in the endothelium (*see* page 25).

Caution: If used in conjunction with Viagra, high doses of L-arginine may cause a drop in blood pressure. And in significant infections there can be an overproduction of NO, causing hypotension (low blood pressure). Dosage should be no more than 3–9 grams daily, in divided doses.

L-Carnitine

L-carnitine is a modified amino acid that helps the body turn fat into energy. It aids in carrying fatty acids into the mitochondria (powerhouse) of the cell. Unless there is sufficient L-carnitine, the body cannot produce enough energy. Producing L-carnitine in the body requires iron, niacin, and vitamins C and B_6. If the blood flow is diminished to the heart muscle, the cause may be insufficient levels of L-carnitine. If levels are low, there will be an accumulation of fatty acids and less energy. Take 1–6 grams daily.

Pregnenelone Hemisuccinate

Pregnenelone hemisuccinate, derived from a naturally occurring steroid, has neuroprotective properties. When neurons die due to a stroke, large amounts of glutamate are released. This causes an activation of N-methyl-D-aspartate (NMDA) receptors from neighboring neurons, which produces more glutamate and the death of more neurons. Receptor blockers, which deactivate excessive glutamate, are well understood. The glutamate attaches to N-methyl receptors, proteins on the cell's surface, in essence preventing glutamate from harming neurons. Since the secondary damage from strokes can be worse than the initial event, pregnenelone hemisuccinate deactivates NMDA receptors, which halt the release of glutamate and confine the secondary damage, so fewer neurons are destroyed. There are currently more than twenty NMDA receptor blockers being tested in clinical studies.

Additional antioxidants protect against brain lesions and lessen the impact of strokes. Although I discuss antioxidants in Chapter 17, the message is worth repeating here, with specific reference to vascular disease.

Vitamin B

Vitamin B_6, B_{12}, and folic acid are homocysteine fighters. Homocysteine is an amino acid (a building block of protein) produced in the body. It can be a blood-vessel irritant helping to create a blockage to blood flow. Homocysteine oxidizes low-density lipoprotein (LDL) to create further blood vessel damage. An elevated homocysteine level encourages heart attacks and strokes. Many heavy meat eaters have elevated homocysteine because meat contains methionine, which is converted to homocysteine and is toxic to the endothelial cell lining of the blood vessels. The standard American diet (SAD) doesn't supply enough B vitamins to detoxify homocysteine. Only a combination of B_6, B_{12}, and folic acid can significantly reduce your homocysteine toxicity level. The goal is a serum level of 8 or less. Recommended dosages include 25 mg of B_6 a day; 100–200 mcg of B_{12} a day; 400–800 mcg of folic acid a day. One product that combines these vitamins, Tri B, is manufactured by Carlson Labs, Arlington Heights, Illinois.

Vitamins C and E

These vitamins can reduce the breakdown of nitrous oxide and enhance arterial relaxation. The Cambridge Heart Antioxidant Study included 2,002 people with known arteriosclerosis. Vitamin E in doses of 400–800 IU decreased the risk of heart attack. I believe that vitamin E is a vital antioxidant and should be a part of your regimen. Take vitamin C in doses of 1,000 mg daily.

Take Note

Physicians who say to an older patient, "You are growing old gracefully" are practicing in the past and are not forward thinkers for enhancing your longevity. And anyone who says eating seven to nine daily servings of fruits and vegetables is sufficient for optimal health is unrealistic. In our hurried, fast-paced, competitive world it would be quite impossible to ingest that many servings of fruits and vegetables, not to mention that quality soil depletion and pollution have lowered the nutrient content of the fruits and vegetables we do consume.

CHAPTER 3

Diseases of the Brain— Alzheimer's Disease

Alzheimer's disease (AD) was discovered in the 1890s by a Geneva physician, Dr. Alois Alzheimer, in the course of treating a fifty-one-year-old patient who had lost her memory. Dr. Alzheimer studied the woman's brain at autopsy, noting different changes with different tissue stains, plaques, and tangles that had never been described before. Other physicians later duplicated his work, but the disease became known as Alzheimer's out of respect for the original doctor.

While we have surpassed all expectations of longevity over the past century—the number of eighty-year-olds is expected to double by 2030 and even triple by 2040—unfortunately, the occurrence of Alzheimer's disease is expected to *triple* over the next forty to fifty years. The financial cost, as well as the emotional impact, is severe.

THE STAGES AND SYMPTOMS OF ALZHEIMER'S DISEASE

Alzheimer's disease is a leading cause of dementia and has predictable stages of impairment.

- **Confusion.** Difficulty in managing activities, such as cleaning, cooking, driving, and shopping.

- **Forgetfulness.** Short-term memory begins to fail and early depression is common (studies have shown that 35 percent of those with AD have significant depression).

- **Inability to communicate reasonably.**

- **Inability to perform such actions as bathing, dressing, and grooming.**

- **Loss of purposeful mobility.**

- **Difficulty managing money.**

Memory loss alone does not mean that you have AD. Depression can cause memory impairment. Low thyroid levels and overmedication can also cause a marked decline in cognition. Multiple TIAs (minor strokes) are also a cause for memory loss, as are vitamin deficiencies due to poor absorption, especially in older patients. Alcoholism is another brain depressor that can result in memory loss.

DIAGNOSING ALZHEIMER'S DISEASE

Today's imaging techniques are very helpful in making accurate diagnoses, which dictate appropriate treatments. However, it is difficult to make a firm diagnosis in someone with early symptoms of dementia because dementia is not a diagnosis, it is a syndrome (a group of signs and symptoms that characterize a particular disease). As with most neurological syndromes, the workup consists of:

- A valid history, not only from the person, but also from family members and friends if possible.

- A physical examination, including mental status. (Who is the president? What is the date?)

- Radiographic studies (MRI, PET, or SPECT).

- Additional laboratory work.

Although new technology can diagnose AD, there is still no standard test to predict who will ultimately get Alzheimer's disease, nor are there any foolproof ways to prevent it. However, early diagnosis allows time to plan for the future and monitor early symptoms. The present drugs available for AD provide symptomatic relief only, and are not long term.

Diagnostic Tools

Positron emission tomography (PET) scanners reveal atrophic (shrunken) areas of the brain indicating Alzheimer's disease. Neil Buckholtz, the dementia chief at the National Institute on Aging, can look at a cross-sectional slice of the brain from the PET scanner and say with certainty whether or not the person has AD.

Single photon emission tomography (SPECT) and PET scans utilize radioactive molecules to determine blood flow and metabolic activity in the brain. People with Alzheimer's disease demonstrate less activity in the temporal and parietal lobes. The newer PET scans are beginning to show the hallmark of the disease—plaques and tangles in the brains of living people.

According to a report at the 103rd Annual Meeting of the American Roentgen Ray Society in 2003, MRIs revealed an increased diffusion of water in the corpus callosum (the band of fibers that unite the cerebral hemispheres), which may correspond to a loss of white-matter cells in that region of the brain.

WHAT CAUSES ALZHEIMER'S DISEASE?

The chief culprit is plaques in the brain, which cause progressive mental loss and destruction. A plaque is a lesion involving brain tissue and consisting of a cluster of degenerating nerve endings around a core of amyloid (protein in combination with polysaccharides). In Alzheimer's, plaques trigger immune cells in the brain, which speeds up the inflammation and the debilitating consequences. New research is aimed at slowing its progression. Nonsteroidal anti-inflammatory drugs (NSAIDs), such as ibuprofen, given to people with rheumatoid arthritis have resulted in a lower incidence of AD in those people. This is because the anti-inflammatory drugs reduce the inflammation caused by the brain's immune cells, which detected and reacted to the amyloid protein as a foreign substance. The inflammatory cells (microglia) activate and secrete toxins, which kill neurons, leading to a loss of memory. Researchers at Case Western Reserve University of Medicine are attempting to block the interaction of the microglia inflammatory cells with the amyloid protein so there would be no inflammatory response and the disease process would be retarded.

The plaques are toxic to brain tissue and cannot be removed by any of the normal metabolic, or clearing, methods. They do their damage by causing interference within the cell and even in the synapse between the cells. The main site for these plaques is the brain's temporal lobes, with progression to the frontal lobes, causing profound memory loss. Another diagnostic brain finding in AD is the tangles. Normally, these axons and dendrites are long branches from the nerve cells (neurons) through which nutrients are transported. In people with Alzheimer's, however, these long threads have become tangles that cannot send nutrients to the nerve endings. As they seem to be found in the temporal lobe first, communication is interrupted. Keep in mind, however, that not all older people with plaques and tangles have AD.

Inflammation of the blood vessels is a major culprit, brought on by plaque. This triggers the inflammatory response, which, in turn, triggers free radicals. The inflammatory process can destroy neurons, and in Alzheimer's, if the repair system is not efficient, the free radicals continue destroying normal neuron cells, leading to a worsening of the Alzheimer's.

Multiple studies have proven that taking supplements with antioxidants, particularly vitamin E, to quench the free radicals is beneficial and therefore recommended. There is another line of thought, however. In numerous studies, autopsies have shown that people with AD didn't always have the dead neurons associated with plaques and tangles.

At the base of the brain, the nucleus basalis of Meynert—a portion of brain matter in the forebrain, which consists mostly of cholinergic neurons—is responsible for producing acetylcholine, an important chemical messenger for communication among neurons. These neurons send their long axon and dendrite branches to the cortex and the hippocampus, the essential part of the brain responsible for forming new memories that lies deep in the brain (subcortical—under the cortex) at the level of your ear canals. If nerve cells die, less acetylcholine reaches the hippocampus, and this causes memory loss. There is a great deal of data to support the idea that atrophy and decreased activity are the primary destructive phenomena in the nucleus basalis of those with Alzheimer's.

Additional studies link elevated homocysteine levels with the risk of AD. In addition, studies at Boston University added a neural-imaging component: Elevated homocysteine levels are toxic and are associated with MRI findings of silent cerebral infarcts (death of tissue) and a change in volume of parts of the brain consistent with AD.

DON'T ASSUME IT'S ALZHEIMER'S DISEASE

Physicians aren't always focused on treatable causes of dementia, but reversing dementia depends on the treatable cause, and AD should not be the initial focus. A mild memory deficit can result from many other conditions, and more than 20 percent of those with a moderate to mild deficit can have a reversible condition, and any reversal equates to the proper diagnosis and

An Alzheimer's Story

Richard, a tenured university professor, decided to retire after his sixtieth birthday to devote his time to writing about philosophy and its history. However, things didn't work out as he had planned. During the last three months of his professorship, he had become very forgetful, and on a few occasions had lost his way on the campus, arriving late for his classes. He forgot a department meeting and didn't show up when scheduled to meet with his students between classes. On one occasion, he had arrived home two hours late for dinner, explaining that his car was out of gas. He had somehow ended up twenty miles away although the school was just three miles from his home.

Because of these problems, Richard's wife brought him to my office for observation and diagnosis. After extensive blood work, which was normal, I had him take his basal axillary temperature for five days upon awakening to rule out hypothyroidism. The temperatures were normal. I then decided to send him for neuropsychological testing. My suspicions were confirmed because the results were very suggestive of Alzheimer's Disease. A PET scan had revealed several areas of atrophy, including both hippocampal structures.

Richard was started on 2,000 IU of vitamin E and an anti-inflammatory. For six months, he was relatively stable, but is now showing signs of depression. His medication has been adjusted, but he has not improved to this point, which, unfortunately, is typical of the 4 million Americans who have this debilitating and progressive brain disorder. It affects 7 percent of the population over the age of sixty-five in the United States, and has devastating effects for those affected, as well as for their families, who may have an even harder time, between taking care of their increasingly dependent loved ones and watching them disintegrate in front of their eyes.

treatment. The most frequent cause of a memory deficit is depression. If you are depressed, you may have difficulty concentrating, and this is followed by forgetfulness. A medical history, a physical exam, blood tests, and imaging studies can decipher this memory conundrum.

Thyroid disease is another cause of forgetfulness. Low-pressure hydrocephalus, caused by an obstruction to the absorption of cerebrospinal fluid, can result in a dementia, a gait (walking) disturbance, or urinary incontinence (all these conditions can be treated with surgical procedures). And certainly alcohol dependence needs to be ruled out.

TREATMENT AND PREVENTION OF ALZHEIMER'S (AD)

The drugs available for AD provide only symptomatic relief. The choline-esterase inhibitors, such as donepezil and tacrine, improve cognition for a while, and can often delay the dreaded nursing home. There are several medications available for the psychiatric manifestations of AD, such as depression, and anti-inflammatory neurotrophic factors and the use of antioxidants—none of which can prevent the disease—are always discussed in connection with AD.

In May 2003, at the 156th Annual Meeting of the American Psychiatric Association, a paper was introduced concerning the benefits of galantamine (Nivalin) treatment for up to forty-eight months in people with mild to moderate Alzheimer's disease. Dr. Mahableshwarker, a researcher at Janssen Pharmaceuticals and an associate professor of psychiatry at the Chicago Medical School, said that even after four years, he continued to see a remarkably diminished decline in patients treated with galantamine (Nivalin). Dr. Aronson, a clinical assistant professor at the University of Michigan Medical School and a researcher of galantamine said, "At this point, the best we can do is slow down the rate of deterioration in patients with AD." His advice to fellow AD therapists was to think of acetylcholinesterase inhibition as an ongoing treatment for stability and for slowing the rate of decline, and to take these results as signs that the person is benefiting from the treatment.

For five to eight years, Martin Rossor and colleagues at the National Hospital in London, followed individuals from a family with a history of an early onset of Alzheimer's disease with known genetic mutations. Four asymptomatic individuals in this family all developed Alzheimer's disease, and were all documented to have a progressive atrophy in specific brain areas before manifesting any disease symptoms. Studies such as these are important because the day will come when scientists will be able to intervene with therapy at the early stage, before an irreversible cognitive decline becomes established.

Vitamins C and D, Folic Acid, and AD

Recent studies have suggested that vitamins C and D might have protective effects against AD. As reported at an annual meeting of the American Academy of Neurology in Honolulu, Hawaii, a high intake of folate (folic acid) is significantly associated with a reduced risk of developing Alzheimer's.

Anti-Inflammatory NSAIDs and AD

Studies of 15,000 AD patients who were prescribed NSAIDs showed a slower progression of the disease. This hypothesis is still under study by the AD Anti-Inflammatory Trial (ADAPT) at six sites in the United States.

Lower Cholesterol and AD

A March 2002 report in the *Archives of Neurology* indicated that high cholesterol might promote the clumping of the beta-amyloid protein, which specifically damages the brain in people with Alzheimer's. The University of California, San Francisco, described the increased risk of cognitive impairment and Alzheimer's disease in a study of older women due to high cholesterol. At the 2002 International Conference on AD in Stockholm, Sweden, lowering cholesterol was thought to reduce AD by 73 percent.

Stress and AD

Susceptibility to psychological distress may be associated with AD. Chronic stress is a link to structural changes in the brain, resulting in impaired memory and learning. "Patients treated for chronic neurosis are prone to an increased risk of AD in the older population," stated Dr. Paul T. Costa, of the National Institute on Aging in Baltimore.

Postcoronary Bypass and AD

Mental impairment is a known risk following coronary bypass surgery. A study reported that the risk of Alzheimer's also increases following bypass surgery. The theory is that the stress induced by the surgery may trigger an increase in the harmful stress hormone cortisol, which could create a cascade of events that led to reduced oxygen to the brain. Neuroprotective drugs, and perhaps increasing glucose to the brain, might have a positive effect.

Genes and AD

Eric M. Reiman at Good Samaritan Regional Medical Center in Phoenix scanned the brains of twelve young people with a known mutation of the APOE gene associated with a high risk of Alzheimer's. They manifested some of the same metabolic changes seen in those who have advanced or mild cases of the disease. This study suggests there are brain changes in people with AD many years before there is an onset of memory loss and cognitive function. Dr. Reiman found that the gene carriers had the abnormally low level of brain glucose metabolism that also occurred in those with diagnosed Alzheimer's. The hope is that earlier intervention might be possible with newer preventive therapies. Parenthetically, it was noted the brains of people affected with HIV contained deposits of the beta-amyloid protein seen in AD.

Statins and AD

In a cardiovascular-health study, people over age sixty-five showed the protective role of statins (anti-cholesterol drugs) against developing AD. When tested by the Modified Mini-Mental Status Exam, the rate of decline in those taking statins was 46 percent lower than the untreated group.

Antioxidants and AD

A recent study reported by Alzheimersupport.com indicated that antioxidant intake is associated with a lower risk for AD. If it is true that oxidative stress involves AD, then antioxidants may well be useful in prevention and treatment.

HRT and AD

A study from Johns Hopkins University in Baltimore, published in the November 6, 2002, issue of *The Journal of the American Medical Association* (*JAMA*) revealed that women who had used hormone replacement therapy (HRT) had a 41 percent reduction in their risk of AD compared to non-HRT users. The result, reported by Peter Zandi, Ph.D., indicates that former users of hormone therapy had a greater reduction in the incidence of AD than those who had not used HRT. Only long-time former users of HRT appeared to have a benefit. Further study of this is underway.

   An alternative conclusion on the value of hormone replacement therapy in AD was put out by Wyeth, the giant drug company that manufactures Prempro (estrogen-progesterone combination). They released a negative state-ment to Reuters News Agency on February 28, 2003, stating that the product may worsen memory among women sixty-five and older. This came about through the study of the Women's Health Initiative, which showed that the drug taken for several years raised the risk for breast carcinoma, heart attacks, and strokes. The new data from Wyeth was from a separate arm of the Women's Health Initiative, and stated that the data showed "negative findings in a small percentage of the study participants." (*See* Chapter 9.)

Vaccines and AD

The promise of a vaccine to treat or prevent AD has been thwarted. Researchers report that in the animal studies, the vaccine cleared the brain of toxic deposits, but doubled the risk of a stroke. There were promising results from a study by the Irish drug company, Elan Corp., in which a beta-amyloid vaccine was used on 360 human test subjects. The clinical trial was suspended because fifteen of them developed an inflammation of the brain tissue. Further, an article in the journal *Science* revealed that another vaccine against beta-amyloid increased bleeding in the brain. An autopsy from a participant in the halted trial showed that although the vaccine cleared the amyloid-beta peptide from most areas of the brain, there was evidence of a meningo-encephalitis, which was considered a direct consequence of the vaccine. Future experiments will hopefully find a successful vaccine.

Although the vaccine study was halted in 2002, Dr. Gilman, a professor of neurology at the University of Michigan, stated at the International Conference on Alzheimer's Disease and Related Disorders in Philadelphia, that the experimental vaccine did show the beta-amyloid clumps had been cleared from the brain tissue. Memory-retention tests demonstrated that the vaccinated group was able to retain memory longer.

Proteins and AD

Scientists at the University of Pennsylvania reported in the April 14, 1993, issue of *The Journal of Cell Biology* that they had found a protein that seals off the mitochondria (powerhouse of the cell) and affects AD neurons, killing the cell. By causing the mitochondria to malfunction, the cell's energy is depleted and it consequently dies.

In the fall of 2003, a new Alzheimer's drug, Memantine, was approved by the FDA for people who have moderately severe to severe Alzheimer's. Used in

Europe for two decades, this drug, which differs from currently available therapies, is the first in a new class specific to AD. This is good news for those in the United States who have AD. Memantine has an affinity for the N-methyl-D-aspartate receptor antagonist (NMDA) and is thought to select and block the excitotoxic effects associated with abnormal transmission of glutamate. For the first time, doctors are able to prescribe combinations of drugs for better results.

The findings of a new study released in 2004 suggest that the drug is effective in all stages of Alzheimer's. The lead investigator, Nunzio Pomara, M.D., a researcher at New York University School of Medicine, said, "Memantine is now our drug of choice in patients who begin to show any signs of mental deterioration." He also added that the Memantine-treated patients were less likely to exhibit agitation or other behavioral disturbances. Its effect is usually apparent after four weeks of treatment.

The drugs being studied are based on the cause and effect of accumulating the beta-amyloid protein in the brain. The approaches to attacking the cause of AD include the removal of accumulated plaque, preventing the formation of such plaques, and interrupting the amyloid precursor protein that initially produces the beta-amyloid.

CHAPTER 4

Diseases of the Brain—
Parkinson's Disease

In 1817, James Parkinson first described Parkinson's disease (PD), the disease subsequently named for him, stating in his monograph:

> After a few more months, the patient is found to be less strict in preserving the upright posture: This being most observable while walking, but sometimes while sitting or standing. Sometime after the appearance of this symptom, and during its slow increase, one of the legs is discovered slightly to tremble, and is also found to suffer fatigue sooner than the leg of the other side. And in a few months this limb becomes agitated by similar tremblings and suffers a similar loss of power.

More than 1.4 million people in the United States have Parkinson's disease, and approximately 50,000 new cases are diagnosed each year. PD is rare in people under age forty; however, 1 percent of the population over age fifty will be diagnosed with it during their lifetimes. In most cases, Parkinson's disease progresses for fifteen to twenty years after the onset of symptoms, although it can reduce life expectancy due to an increased infection rate caused by chronic immobility.

CAUSES OF PARKINSON'S DISEASE

The cause of Parkinson's disease is unknown, nor is it known how the specific neurons become impaired. Research suggests a genetic component, especially in early onset, and this is found more in women than men. Most people with Parkinson's do not have a definitive genetic abnormality.

External and Internal Environmental Factors and PD

Research at the Mayo Clinic in Rochester, Minnesota, suggests that environmental factors play a greater role in the development of PD in men, and hereditary factors play a greater role for women.

"For women, genetic predisposition may be more important because they are less exposed to environmental risk factors linked to PD in previous research," said Dr. Demetrius Maraganore, a Mayo Clinic neurologist involved in the study. "Also estrogen may protect women's brains from the effect of these environmental factors."

Environmental toxins—herbicides, industrial chemicals, and pesticides—can selectively destroy the dopaminergic neuron, thereby causing Parkinson's. The toxins include carbon disulfide, carbon monoxide, and manganese, which cause oxidative damage to the substantia nigra. Many autopsy studies indicate that free radicals cause the damage.

An increase in brain-iron content is probably due to oxidation and the subsequent production of free radicals. Autopsies have shown a diminished glutathione level in the brains of people with Parkinson's, which indicates a breakdown of the antioxidant protection system.

The midbrain area known as the substantia nigra is pigmented matter containing cells that produce the neurotransmitter dopamine. The substan-

Toxic Manganese

In my practice, I have seen toxic exposure to manganese cause a Parkinsonian syndrome. John, a welder, was unknowingly exposed to manganese in the air at a smelter, caused by a malfunctioning ventilation system. The exposure was for only a week, one to two hours a day, but it was sufficient time for him to develop muscle stiffness, slow movement, and tremors, with his muscle rigidity leading to poor balance and difficulty walking.

Even though the malfunctioning ventilation system was repaired and his blood and urine levels returned to normal, his condition has continued to progress over the last five years, and hair analysis reveals that there are still traces of manganese in his body. Manganese levels are high in the production of batteries, ceramics, fertilizers, and pesticides, and anyone working with large-scale amounts of these products should be tested if they show any symptoms of Parkinson's.

tia nigra is rich in melatonin, a precursor to dopamine. It produces the chemical messenger involved in the communication between the corpus striatum (a pair of nerve-tissue masses on the floor of the brain with nuclei separated by sheets of white matter in the substantia nigra).

This relationship produces smooth, balanced muscle movement. A deficiency of dopamine results in the abnormal nerve functioning that causes loss of control in body movements. By the time symptoms develop, there may be an 80 to 90 percent loss of the dopamine-producing cells.

Drug Factors and PD

An illegal, street-synthesized form of heroin (N-MPTP) can cause Parkinson's disease, which is not reversible following the drug's discontinuance. Some antipsychotic drugs that treat paranoia and schizophrenia can cause symptoms resembling Parkinson's disease, but these are usually reversible after the drugs are discontinued.

Additional drugs known to worsen symptoms of PD are Reserpine, a diuretic; antipsychotics, such as chlorpromazine; and Verapamil, a heart drug. Naproxen and other nonsteroidal anti-inflammatory drugs (NSAIDs) may also exacerbate Parkinson's.

Other Diseases, Neurotoxic Events, and PD

Other diseases, such as arteriosclerosis or strokes, can cause symptoms similar to PD, and a prior neurotoxic event may cause symptoms similar to it. Research in Iceland, which has a high incidence of PD, showed that children born during or after a whooping-cough epidemic are particularly prone to PD later in life. This suggests that a neurotoxic event, which occurred at an early age, may influence the occurrence of PD later in life.

Trauma and PD

A recent study published in *The Journal of Neurology* suggests that head trauma, even twenty years prior to the onset of Parkinson's, may be the contributing factor for some cases of PD. A study at the Mayo Clinic in Rochester, Minnesota, found that a minor head injury without loss of consciousness did not increase the risk, but people who had experienced a serious head trauma had an eleven times higher risk for developing PD years later. Hundreds of boxers, along with their medical histories, were reviewed for this study.

Free-Radical Destruction and PD

What causes the destruction of the dopamine-producing cells is still unknown, but more of a consensus is emerging that the cause is oxidative stress (free-radical destruction). In 1994, two professors at King's College, London, proposed that neurodegenerative diseases, and Parkinson's in particular, were the result of oxidative stress.

Many studies have shown that people with PD have low levels of the natural antioxidants superoxide dismutase and glutathione. There are also high levels of iron in the substantia nigra area, which are thought to help catalyze free radicals into destroying the dopamine-producing cells. Several similar metals, such as cadmium, copper, manganese, and mercury (from dental amalgams), have been implicated in the development of Parkinson's. High aluminum levels in drinking water have also been associated with an excessive risk of developing PD.

SYMPTOMS OF PARKINSON'S DISEASE

A tremor is an involuntary movement that may affect the limbs, head, or entire body, but is most prominent in the fingers and hands. The movement is most visual when the person is at rest and it may increase with stress. During sleep, the tremor ceases.

Postural instability is characterized by a deteriorating ability to write, and a decreased arm swing when walking. The person's posture gradually stoops, progressing to flexed knees and a toe-first walk.

Bradykinesia (slowness of movement) may be the most disabling feature, where there is a lack of facial expression and slowness in chewing, eating, and eye blinking. Rigidity in some is characterized by stiffness and an increase in poor muscle tone affecting both the flexor and extensor muscle groups, with difficulty initiating any movement, such as getting up from a chair. This can be interrupted by brief relaxations, primarily in the hands, when the tremor is at rest.

Depression is common in the early stages of Parkinson's, and interestingly, up to 30 percent of those with PD eventually develop Alzheimer's disease or other forms of dementia.

TREATMENTS FOR PARKINSON'S DISEASE

An expanding awareness of alternative treatments has led to a number of ways to treat this debilitating disease.

Supplements and PD

Antioxidants are required to quench free radicals caused by oxidative damage. In 1991, Dr. Stanley Fahn of Columbia University in New York did a study demonstrating that antioxidants slow down the progression of existing PD. In the test group diagnosed with Parkinson's, but not needing conventional prescription medication, those taking antioxidants had an extended time frame and did not need prescribed drugs for an additional 2.5 years. The results indicated the importance of the antioxidants in slowing the progression of PD.

Acetyl-L-Carnitine and PD

Acetyl-L-carnitine is an important factor in the transfer of long-chain fatty acids across the mitochondrial membrane. It also is involved in the formation of acetylcholine, the important neurotransmitter, and is a superior antioxidant in enhancing energy production in damaged neurons.

Coenzyme Q_{10} and PD

Coenzyme Q_{10} (ubiquinone) slows the progression of Parkinson's. A study cited in the *Archives of Neurology* suggested a slower rate of deterioration in patients.

"Tissue CoQ_{10} levels fall with aging and we do not know why this occurs," said Richard Haas, M.D., an investigator at the University of California, San Diego, who described the results of the study. "The normal lower levels of CoQ_{10} in older individuals may be a contributing factor in the progression of some diseases of aging."

The most dramatic effects in people with Parkinson's were apparent in daily activities, including bathing, dressing, feeding, and walking. Those who were taking 1,200 mg of CoQ_{10} per day showed a 44 percent slower deterioration than those in the placebo group.

Note. Statin drugs, used for lowering cholesterol, also lowers serum CoQ_{10} levels.

Flavonoids and PD

Because flavonoids, particularly grapeseed and pine-bark extract, are water soluble and can readily cross the blood-brain barrier, it is easier to deliver the

The Blood-Brain Barrier (BBB)

This semi-permeable membrane allows some molecules to cross into the brain, while excluding others. The primary purpose of the BBB is to maintain a constant environment and keep out any foreign substances that would injure the brain. This valuable, intact safety system is threatened by brain trauma, hypertension, infections, inflammation, ischemia, microwaves, radiation, or a rush of highly concentrated toxins in the blood.

benefits of these important antioxidants to the brain. Neuroprotective flavonoids, present in a diet of fruit peelings, have the ability to chelate (bind) metal ions and remove them from the body.

Ginkgo Biloba and PD

Ginkgo biloba increases blood flow to the brain, and studies on lab animals have shown it to be protective in the development of Parkinson's disease. It is known to enhance and preserve cognitive performance, and should therefore be included here. It is also effective in the treatment of Alzheimer's disease.

Glutathione and PD

Glutathione is a most important brain chemical and antioxidant, and PD patients have a profound deficiency of this chemical. Beyond glutathione's role as a major antioxidant, it recycles vitamins C and E. Dr. David Perlmutter, the author of brainrecovery.com has been using glutathione IV since 1998 for people with Parkinson's, and these people show "profound improvements with respect to reduction of rigidity, increased mobility, improved ability to speak, less depression and decreased tremor." Although glutathione declines with age, higher levels are associated with better health.

Liver detoxification is important since there may be a flaw in the liver's ability to detoxify many chemicals. By giving glutathione, both the liver and brain are detoxified.

N-Acetyl-L-Cystine and PD

N-acetyl-L-cystine, a potent antioxidant, enhances glutathione production in the brain. For this to occur successfully, vitamin C must be added.

NADH and PD

NADH (nicotinamide adenine dinucleotide) is an enzyme that helps produce energy in living cells, particularly in the brain. Original work by Dr. Jorg Birkmayer in 1993 revealed that 80 percent of 885 test subjects with Parkinson's who received NADH had a moderate to excellent improvement in their disabilities. NADH enhanced the production of dopamine and neuroadrenaline, and also increased energy production in brain cells.

Phosphatidylserine and PD

Phosphatidylserine (PS), an important component of the neuronal membrane, can enhance the production of dopamine. The mitochondrial membrane is composed of PS, which needs to be boosted to maintain normal functioning.

Vitamin C and PD

Vitamin C does not naturally cross the blood-brain barrier, but it does enter the cerebrospinal fluid that bathes the brain, and it quenches the free radicals that are the main destroyers of the dopamine cell.

Vitamin E and PD

Vitamin E is a fat-soluble vitamin that does not readily cross the blood-brain barrier. However, when taken in high doses, it is found in the brain. As an antioxidant that acts in the fatty parts of cells and nerve tissue, it stops the chain reaction of free radicals by surrendering its own electron, thereby protecting healthy molecules from harm. Nevertheless, studies conflict on its actual value in the treatment of PD.

Other recommended treatments include those listed below.

Animal Fats and PD

A high intake of animal fats is associated with five times greater occurrence or risk of developing PD. It is therefore important to restrict the intake of meats, which are high in saturated fats.

Calorie Restriction and PD

Calorie restriction in relationship to neurodegenerative disorders has been studied at the University of Kentucky Medical Center. Mark Mattson, Ph.D., a professor of anatomy and neurobiology, who did an extensive study in rats, said, "The importance of these studies is that food restriction can reduce the vulnerability of new cells in the brain to insults relevant to several different human age-related disorders. . . . Formal studies of calorie intake and neurodegenerative disorders have not been performed in humans, but there appears to be a strong correlation between per-capita food intake and the incidence of age-related neurodegenerative disorders."

While there is no cure yet for Parkinson's disease, research is dedicated to lowering the risk of developing it. Along with calorie restriction, the best preventive therapy involves reducing or eliminating the intake of animal fats and sugar, consuming a diet rich in fruits and vegetables, avoiding exposure to toxic metals, and assuring an optimum intake of antioxidants. Dosages should be discussed with a nutritionally aware healthcare professional.

Conventional Treatments and PD

The neurotransmitter dopamine, NPD, does not pass through the blood-brain barrier and most doctors will prescribe a regimen of drugs, such as L-dopa or Sinemet, that can cross the BBB and convert into dopamine within the brain. L-dopa medications bring significant relief from Parkinson's, but they become less effective over time and require increasing dosage, with the effect less predictable. As PD progresses, depression increases and may need to be treated. Just as statin drugs (cholesterol-lowering drugs) wash out CoQ_{10}, L-dopa medications may lead to a vitamin-B deficiency, primarily of niacin and B_6. The recommendation for L-dopa is to delay starting it as long as possible after the diagnosis in order to postpone the adverse effects.

The medications available to battle the progression of Parkinson's should be managed by a neurologist well trained in movement disorders. A combination of drugs and dosages are individually selected, and it may take trial and error to determine what is optimum for each person.

Complementary Treatments and PD

Complementary treatments include CoQ_{10} and anthocyanidins (grapeseed extracts, bilberry). This group has up to fifty times more potency than vitamin

E and can readily cross the blood-brain barrier to perform free-radical-scavenging action. Stress can aggravate PD. Relaxation therapies, physical therapy, and exercise can help moderate the disease.

Surgical Treatments and PD

Most people with Parkinson's are treated with medications to alleviate their symptoms. However, in 15 to 20 percent of the cases, medications are not sufficiently effective and surgical treatment may be an option.

Surgical approaches include:

- **Deep-brain stimulation.** There is no destruction of brain tissue in this new procedure in which electrodes are placed in the thalamus or the globus pallidus and connected to a pacemaker device (an impulse generator), which is implanted under the skin beneath the collarbone. The device sends a continuous electrical impulse to the brain target, which blocks the tremors. These stimulators can last three to five years and are programmed with a computer that sends signals to the impulse generator.

- **Pallidotomy.** In PD, a part of the brain called the globus pallidus becomes overactive and creates a problem with bodily movement. The surgical goal is to destroy this area in order to aid in balance, lessen the symptoms of rigidity, and reduce tremors.

- **Subthalamic nucleus stimulation.** This newest procedure in the deep-brain stimulation technique can address the full gamut of Parkinson's symptoms—rigidity, slow movement, and tremors. If successful, the individual may be able to reduce her or his medications. Overall, deep-brain stimulation has fewer complications than a thalamotomy or a pallidotomy, and does not require destruction of brain tissue. The strength of electrical stimulation can be adjusted to the individual patient. The 2 to 3 percent risk of serious complications includes a change in memory or personality and the chance that seizures may occur.

- **Thalamotomy.** The abnormal brain activity that causes tremors is processed through the thalamus. This procedure destroys part of the thalamus, blocking the abnormal brain activity, which otherwise would reach the muscles and cause the often severe tremor. This procedure reduces the intensity of, but does not eliminate, the tremors.

People who do not achieve satisfactory control with medications may become candidates for invasive or surgical procedures of this type. In cases reported by Stanford University, surgery has improved symptoms by as much as 85 percent.

ONGOING AND FUTURE RESEARCH

Parkinson's has no shortage of research connected to it, and some seems most promising.

Clioquinol

Clioquinol, a known antibiotic and methyl chelator (derived from the Greek word for claw), is being investigated at the Buck Institute in Novato, California, to remove excessive iron from brain cells. Binding the iron and removing it stops the oxidation process, which can damage the neurons of the substantia nigra area of the brain. These studies were successful in mice and may lead to human trials.

Fetal Cell Transplantation

Fetal cells are implanted into the brain to replace the deficient dopamine-producing cells within the substantia nigra. This is controversial. There have been cases where stem-cell fetal-cell transplantation has caused an increase in involuntary movement because there was too much dopamine. There also are objections to the procedure on moral and ethical grounds.

Glial Cell-Line-Derived Neurotrophic Factor (GDNF)

This is a new treatment being investigated by Clive N. Svendse at the University of Wisconsin, Madison. The online journal *Nature Medicine* reported that the new bioengineered medication positively affected the five people tested. The trial consists of implanting a miniature battery-driven pump under the skin overlying the chest. A tube is placed into the area of the substantia nigra in the brain and is connected to the pump, which delivers a continuous dose of GDNF. To date, the results suggest that GDNF has protected the cells from damage, and has helped to actually regenerate some of the damaged cells. Dr. Svendse, who followed these people for two years, says they remain free of any side effects.

Homocysteine Levels

A study at the University of Texas Southwestern Medical Center in Dallas revealed how it was not uncommon to see people with Parkinson's who took L-dopa develop elevated homocysteine levels, and subsequently heart disease. Anyone with Parkinson's should be tested and treated for elevated homocysteine levels.

L-Dopa (Levodopa)

This drug converts into dopamine in the brain, but to achieve the optimum benefit, two other substances, carbidopa and entacapone, are added to the same pill. These inhibit enzymes that help degrade the L-dopa and allow for a greater and more continuous delivery. By extending its half-life, the person can remain active longer between doses.

Neural Growth Factor

These combination chemicals may provide stimulation for dopamine production. Research is ongoing.

Newer Drug Treatment

Studies are currently underway to find a drug to block the action of glutamate, an amino acid known to destroy cells. CoQ_{10} has recently been added to the regimen to slow the progression of PD. Glutamate is an excitotoxin, and excess glutamate can overstimulate nerve cells to their death if unopposed. This event can be offset by CoQ_{10}, which helps turn glucose (blood sugar) into energy in all cells of the body. If, however, the body lacks sufficient levels of CoQ_{10} to oppose the excess glutamate, the nerve cells will exhaust themselves and die.

Stalevo

This recently released drug allows people with PD to have better control over their symptoms. It is more convenient to administer this triple combination drug than the standard therapy. Levodopa has been a mainstay drug for PD, but after one or two years of use, its beneficial effects wear off. Stalevo is designed to be delivered to the brain at a steadier level, thereby extending the control for longer periods of time each day and significantly improving the ability to control PD. Stalevo is a combination of three drugs in one pill—Entacapone, carbidopa, and levodopa.

Stem Cell Transplantation

Stem cells are the parent cells of all the tissues in the body and can mature into any type of cell—that is, there is a stem cell for every type of cell. Research continues on the process of turning stem cells into specific cells that will create dopamine-producing neurons, but there is a risk of overproducing dopamine. Gene therapy is currently the best hope that specific, coded proteins can be utilized to produce dopamine.

Testosterone

A report from the 54th Annual Meeting of the American Academy of Neurology in Denver, Colorado, in April 2002 discussed the deficiency of testosterone in men with Parkinson's. This deficiency accounts for several important nonmotor symptoms, such as anxiety, a decrease in libido, and depression. Testosterone replacement has made a significant improvement in people with PD.

CHAPTER 5

The Brainpower Risk-Assessment Test

The ancestor of every action is a thought.

—EMERSON

While treating patients in my private practice, an unexpected and repetitious medical pattern emerged. It became starkly apparent that many of them were deficient in certain hormones and neurotransmitters. There were observably clear differences in the patients' mental, physical, and emotional well-being. Their imbalances were not from external factors, such as drug addiction or life-threatening diseases, but rather from internal ones, such as hormone depletion and decline. Simply put, this is why people age.

Everyone ages differently. Physicians need to recognize that aging is a depletion process. Diet, gender, genetics, lifestyle choices, mental stimulation, metabolism, and yes, age, have to be factored into any successful probrain and age-management program.

The need for a personalized approach to my patients' health led me to develop a risk-assessment test. This is an easy-to-complete questionnaire based on years and thousands of hours interfacing with my patients. The results will be a blueprint for your Brainpower regimen, with guidelines on diet, exercise, medications, and supplements. Before embarking on any major change in diet, exercise, nutritional supplements, or even medications, you should know exactly what your health status is at this moment.

The best way to maximize the results of your regimen is by consulting a knowledgeable, nutritionally-aware healthcare professional. Although this book is one of the first to focus on the brain as the most important organ in the aging process, you need a complete medical history, as well as a physical and laboratory evaluation. If you are taking any medications, ask about recommended supplements, as they might conflict chemically.

Before we begin, it is useful to briefly review some pertinent statistics about the three leading causes of brain disease:

- After age sixty-five, the incidence of Alzheimer's disease doubles every five years.

- By age eighty-five, you have more than a 50 percent chance of being hypertensive. This is a precursor to stroke, which affects more than 50 million Americans. There are 750,000 new strokes each year, and hypertension is the culprit in 50 percent of those cases.

- The incidence of Parkinson's disease is increasing. It now affects 15 percent of those between ages sixty-five and seventy-six, and 30 percent of those seventy-five to eighty-five.

Anti-aging research, medical and complementary, has given us an alternative array of preventive methods to combat these enemies of brain health. Now it is time to know more about what makes you tick—your strengths and your weaknesses—in the battle for brain health. This questionnaire will take ten minutes to complete. It is designed to assess your risks for the three leading causes of brain disease listed above. Be unflinchingly honest in your answers. Later in the book you'll learn how to build a personalized brain-health regimen for your age group.

PART I. ALZHEIMER'S RISK FACTOR

1. Does your family have a history of Alzheimer's disease before age sixty-five? If yes, record 4 points. After age sixty-five? If yes, record 3 points. _____

2. Have you ever had multiple head injuries? If yes, add 2 points. _____

3. Have you had any inflammation of the brain, such as encephalitis? If yes, add 2 points. _____

4. Are you using aluminum utensils and/or antacids such as Alternagel? If yes, add 2 points. _____

5. Do you have ongoing food allergies or other allergies in general? If yes, add 2 points. _____

6. Are you exposed to metals: lead, mercury, or cadmium (acrylic paints)? If yes, add 3 points. _____

7. Do you have elevated blood levels of homocysteine? If yes, add 3 points. _____

8. Are you a woman not taking estrogen replacement therapy (HRT), despite loss of ovarian function from menopause, surgery, or other causes? If yes, add 3 points. _____

9. If you are a woman, add 2 points. _____

10. Do you have poor memory retention? Do you often forget what you did or what you were going to do in ten minutes or less? If yes, add 2 points. _____

11. Did you have difficulty graduating from high school because of poor retention? If yes, add 1 point. _____

12. Is it difficult to follow a plot in a television show or a movie? If yes, add 2 points. _____

13. Do you have difficulty doing mathematical skills: paying bills or balancing a checkbook? If yes, add 2 points. _____

Alzheimer's Risk Factor (continued)

14. Have people close to you said you're not yourself? Do you have personality changes? If yes, add 1 point.   _____

15. Is it difficult to understand or remember something you've just read? If yes, add 2 points.   _____

16. Do you forget where you are going and get lost frequently? If yes, add 2 points.   _____

17. Is it harder to learn new things? If yes, add 2 points.   _____

18. Have friends commented that you seem moody, irritable, or less interested? If yes, add 1 point.   _____

19. Are you indecisive? Is it harder to reach decisions about simple matters? If yes, add 1 point.   _____

20. Do you feel a decline in the ability to form new ideas or think creatively? If yes, add 2 points.   _____

21. Has anyone told you that your memory is getting worse? If yes, add 2 points.   _____

Add up your total number of points and record it here: _____

For this part, you will need a pen and a timepiece with a secondhand.

1. Name ten types of birds in two minutes or less.

   Score 1 point if you wrote fewer than ten.
   Score 2 points if you wrote fewer than five.

Record your score here: _____

Total score for the Alzheimer's factor: _____

PART II. PARKINSON'S RISK FACTOR

1. Do you have a family history of Parkinson's disease?
   If yes, record 4 points. _____

2. If you are a man, add 3 points. _____

3. Do you feel an overall slowing of movement?
   If yes, add 2 points. _____

4. Looking into a mirror, does your face lack emotion?
   Is it vacant? If yes, add 2 points. _____

5. Do you feel tired and listless most of the time?
   If yes, add 1 point. _____

6. Is it difficult to initiate new projects? If yes, add 2 points. _____

7. Are emotional events difficult for you to respond or
   relate to? If yes, add 1 point. _____

8. Do you lose balance, stumble, or bump into things
   more than ever? If yes, add 2 points. _____

9. Take these quick dexterity tests: If your actions are
   rapid, score 0. If you are slow, score 4 points.

   a) Tap your thumb against your index finger
      (very fast) ten times. _____

   b) Open your hand as wide as you can and close
      it rapidly ten times. _____

10. Is your sexual interest diminished? If yes, add 1 point. _____

11. Examine your posture. While walking ask a friend to observe.

    a) Is your posture stooped forward or veering off to
       one side? If yes, add 3 points. _____

    b) Do you walk with short shuffling steps? If yes,
       add 3 points. _____

    c) While walking, are your arms swinging out from
       your body? If not, add 2 points. _____

Parkinson's Risk Factor (continued)

12. Are your arms or legs rigid or stiff when you move them? If yes, add 2 points. _____

13. Do your hands or fingers move involuntarily? Do you have tremors or shaking while at rest? If yes to either, add 3 points for each. _____

14. Have your muscles grown weaker? Do you drop things often? Is lifting or picking up more difficult? If yes to any of these, add 1 point for each. _____

15. Has your reaction time decreased, as, for example, when driving? If yes, add 1 point. _____

16. Is your speech tone flatter or a monotone (you can ask a friend to help you answer this). If yes, add 2 points. _____

17. Is there a general lack of emotion toward people, including family? If yes, add 1 point. _____

18. Do you find it difficult to wake up or stay alert after drinking caffeinated drinks? Does it take two or more cups to stay alert? If yes, add 1 point. _____

19. Do you cook with iron pots and pans? If yes, add 2 points. _____

20. Do you take vitamins with iron (Geritol, for example)? If yes, add 2 points. _____

21. Is it difficult to start or initiate movements of your body? If yes, add 3 points. _____

22. Are you or have you ever been exposed to pesticides? If yes, add 3 points. _____

Total score for the Parkinson's factor: _____

PART III. STROKE RISK FACTOR

1. Do you have a family history of stroke? If yes, record 4 points. _____

2. Do you smoke? If yes, add 3 points. _____

3. Do you smoke at least a pack of cigarettes a day? If yes, add 4 points. _____

4. Do you live with someone who smokes? If yes, add 1 point. _____

5. Are you hypertensive? If yes, add 4 points. _____

6. Do you have episodes of irritability, aggressiveness, or losing your temper? If yes, add 2 points. _____

7. Do you need drugs or alcohol to relax from a stressful day more than occasionally? If yes, add 3 points. _____

8. Do you tend to be obsessive/compulsive in daily habits, which bothers you or others? If yes, add 2 points. _____

9. Is your LDL (bad) cholesterol level above normal limits? If yes, add 3 points. _____

10. Have you been diagnosed with diabetes? If yes, add 3 points. _____

11. Are you clinically obese? (*See* Chapter 11—body mass index) If yes, add 2 points. _____

12. Are you a man? If yes, add 2 points. _____

13. Are you an African American? If yes, add 1 point. _____

14. Do you eat fish less than once a month? If yes, add 2 points. _____

15. Do you have insomnia, or take hours to fall asleep and stay asleep? If yes, add 2 points. _____

16. Do you exercise at least thirty minutes, three times a week? If no, add 3 points. _____

Total score for the stroke factor: _____

HOW TO INTERPRET YOUR SCORES

Compare the total scores for each of the three sections of the test. The section with the highest score determines which of the three major dangers to your brain health you are at highest risk for. For example, if the highest of your three scores is for the Parkinson's test, that means of the three most prevalent pro-aging brain conditions, you are at risk for Parkinson's disease to some degree. Assessing your risk is the first step in building your personalized Brainpower regimen. In subsequent chapters, you will learn about the next steps for prolonging your life and the health of your brain. Remember this assessment is only a guide and may not be statistically valid.

CHAPTER 6

Your Nutritional Defense: Five Super Strategies for Brain Health

Let food be thy medicine.

—HIPPOCRATES

From the time of the ancients, we have known that diet plays an enormous role in the state of our health. The original visionary was Hippocrates, the father of medicine, who counseled his fellow Greeks on the value of a natural diet. From the earliest recorded times, whole foods were heralded, and honored, by physicians and their patients.

In the 1950s, Adele Davis, who pioneered the discussion of nutrition in American homes, said, "As I see it, every day you can do one of two things: build health or produce disease in yourself." Some of her advice is still valid. Her most important contribution was a continual endorsement of unprocessed foods, which even in the 1950s, began to be replaced on grocery shelves by frozen and preservative-laden products. Davis was ahead of her time because, in the last few decades, these chemical additives have become the most prevalent factors in brain disease. The occurrence of degenerative brain disease is now greater than at any other time in the history of humankind.

WHAT YOU EAT IS A STATE OF MIND

Research has shown that it is possible to improve your mental health by eating healthier foods. A Capital Food and Mood project based in Great Britain has shown that what we eat has a significant effect on our state of mind. Two hundred participants in this study cut down on *food stressors,* such as alcohol, caffeine, chocolate, and sugar, and increased the *supporters,* which included water, fruits, vegetables, and oily fish. They had to eat regularly and not skip breakfast, and 88 percent of them remarked that changing to this diet significantly improved their mental health. Twenty-six percent reported feeling less depressed. More than one-third of the participants were "very certain" that the improvements they saw in their mental health were directly linked to the changes they made in their diet.

FOODS OF THE FORAGERS

Our hunting and gathering ancestors were living proof of the merits of a high-protein diet. It was imperative to have the strength and energy to go out daily and forage for survival, and this need to bring in food every day motivated and exercised their minds and bodies. In this effort, they ate fresh, unprocessed, and undercooked plant and animal foods, which for them had the highest energy value and were the very best for their harsh existence. In this lifestyle, they metabolized foods more efficiently than people do today, in large part because there wasn't any food industry around to process or corrupt the vital seeds of nutrient energy. This history is relevant to anyone alive today, for unless you maintain a garden, and/or hunt for your meat, most of your foods must be purchased from the grocery shelves. And most of these are intentionally processed for a long shelf-life, which is most likely what you are ingesting—foods that are developed primarily for shelf life instead of nutritive value.

With the invention of milling, foods became the overprocessed grains and nutrients that we see and eat today. For foods to last longer on the shelves, they were separated (purposely) from their original nutrient source, which devalued most, if not all, the energy of the food. Bread was originally made with whole grains and was far mealier than the highest-fiber bread of today. That was when *stoneground* meant just that, before the advent of the over-processed, chemical-laden foods that we consume today.

It has been proven over and over that present-day diets and the lifestyles of most people today are worlds away from the foods that our ancestors consumed. It is also vastly different from any of the societies that still eat as their ancestors did, people such as those in sub-Saharan Africa, with their fiber and grain-rich diets. Sadly, in just fifty years, an untold number of chemicals, preservatives, and other additives have been embedded in the food supply, and the effect on good health has been devastating, as people are just beginning to realize, with cancer, diabetes, and obesity, for example, becoming epidemic.

THE FOLLY OF THE FDA

A popular ice cream brand has used a brilliant marketing strategy for many years: A precocious child reads the list of ingredients from its competitors' products and then compares the list of natural foodstuffs that go into its own product. It's a common tactic aimed at those who peruse the side panels of American manufactured food. "But it *has* to be safe," many of my patients protest. "It's been approved by the FDA." This rational point of view is, unfortunately, a misinformed one. It makes sense that this mammoth agency's primary task would be to protect the food (both natural and processed varieties) of the American people. But is it true? Indeed, no. Tens of thousands of lobbyists, with profit instead of the best and safest nutrition on their minds, wine, dine, and otherwise cajole policymakers in the hope of gaining FDA approval for their *advanced* chemical compounds and additive-dependent manufacturing processes—and they succeed. A quick look at the ingredients of most packaged foods is proof positive of this incontrovertible fact.

Some of my patients say they don't understand what these chemicals are, and can't even pronounce them, but go on to say, "Still, they have to be safe—or, at least, benign—or they would never be approved by the FDA, right?" To which I have to respond, "Wrong." And why? Because one man's approval is another man's gimmick in the deliberate semantic confusion indulged in by the food industry. Using words as a smokescreen to the public has become the large-scale ruination of American health and, more specifically, the health of people's brains. There is an increasing amount of scientific proof that food additives cause impairments in the brain's health and functioning.

THE SHELF-LIFE SCANDAL

How did harmful additives come to inhabit the aisles of North American supermarkets and, increasingly, those of the rest of the world? It is because food manufacturers are interested in shelf life and not your life. If this sounds like a searing indictment of the American food industry, that's exactly what it is.

It is time to face reality and learn how these companies keep potentially lifesaving information from the public at large. They do it through their lobbyists and public relations firms, who use their influence with the FDA. As the insurance company commercial goes, "They have lawyers on their side . . . and so should you." Awareness of the dangers of the current food and agribusiness industry and advocating for food with health benefits are what I preach to my patients.

The intent of this book is to cause a change in the eating habits of people everywhere and make them aware of the villains that exist on the grocery shelves. You must make healthier food choices. Be diligent.

THE FOOD FOES YOU MUST KNOW

Food does not always feed the mind; sometimes, it destroys it. In fact, there is voluminous scientific evidence that many common chemical additives in prepared, store-bought foods cause brain damage in both children and adults over time. It is an insidious process.

I believe these additives can explain the huge number of children with attention-deficit disorder, behavioral dysfunctions, other learning disabilities, and even emotional disorders, which were undetectable before the processed-food generation. In adults, these chemical additives can cause disorders ranging from memory loss and emotional problems, referred to as chemical imbalances in the brain, to malignant tumors of the brain. Yes, brain tumors.

Chemicals, including aspartame (the most widely ingested sugar substitutes—Nutrasweet and Equal sweeteners—are as addictive as sugar) and monosodium glutamate (MSG), found in much more than just Chinese food, are basically contained in all processed foods. And all these foods have been shown to produce neurodegenerative brain diseases, such as Alzheimer's; amyotrophic lateral sclerosis (ALS), known as Lou Gehrig's disease; Parkinson's; and even strokes (brain attacks).

EXCITOTOXINS—CHEMICAL WARFARE IN YOUR BRAIN

Why the excitement over the excitotoxins? Science has shown that excitotoxin compounds in your foods play a critical role in the development of neurological disorders, which include endocrine disruption, learning disabilities, migraines, neural defects in the fetus, seizures, and others. The year-by-year increase in these additives, and the damage they do, is still refuted by the FDA and the food industry.

The initial marketing of these products indicated the use of additives for the preservation of foods. However, they never had anything to do with protecting the integrity of food; their job is to alter the taste of foods. They have all been introduced in order to enhance taste and magnify a desired, even addictive, taste.

These chemical brain foes have recently been named excitotoxins by the scientific community, and were so named because these manufactured substances exist solely to *excite* our taste buds and create an ongoing desire for them. As they do so, however, they overstimulate the sensitive brain neurons and eventually end up burning them out completely. The primary excitotoxins, aspartame and MSG, are particularly insidious because the way they work is not detectable. By the time their cumulative action is done, it may be too late.

These ubiquitous excitotoxins are disguised by innocuous-sounding names, such as aspartame, caseinate, hydrolyzed vegetable protein, MSG, natural flavorings, soy protein extract, textured protein, and vegetable protein. Liquid excitotoxins in diet sodas, soups, and gravies are more toxic than those added to solid foods because liquid is more rapidly absorbed and reaches the bloodstream faster, causing higher blood levels in a shorter time.

An excitotoxin starts out as an acidic amino acid, which reacts with a specialized brain cell receptor, and can lead to the destruction of those cells. The effects of most excitotoxins are slow, although in hypersensitive individuals, symptoms can develop rapidly or acutely.

There are more than seventy known excitotoxins, including MSG, the sodium salt of glutamate. Glutamate by itself is a normal neurotransmitter in the brain that, in lower concentrations, is found on the outside of the cell. Why is it damaging then? Because when it's increased in concentrations that cause neurons to fire in an abnormal way, it encourages a delayed cellular death.

California, Pizza, and MSG

On a trip to California with my wife and children several years ago, we stopped for pizza at a well-known chain. As she always does, my wife asked about MSG in the pizza sauce and got the standard answer, "Oh no, it's all natural and fresh." As we began eating our slices, my wife began to cough and sneeze uncontrollably and her eyes were watering heavily. Before I knew it, she had run out of the restaurant, and it had all happened within thirty to forty seconds of her first bite of pizza.

Outside, I saw she had difficulty getting her breath, but the fresh air helped stop her acute tracheal spasms and allowed her breathing to return to normal. Being in excellent health—even though ultrasensitive to a noxious food additive—my wife was able to weather the event. But what about those people whose health is frail? It could be disastrous for them.

When glutamate combines with other excitatory amino acids to open the calcium channel on the membrane of the nerve cell, another negative chemical reaction can occur, which allows excess calcium to enter the cell. When the calcium in the cell causes excess firing of impulses, this, in turn, causes free-radical production, lipid peroxidation, and cellular death (excitotoxic reaction). When these brain cells are damaged or destroyed, the release of glutamate from the surrounding cells causes further damage to normal nerves and the result is trauma to the brain and strokes.

The accumulation of these food-borne toxins adds to brain damage. Many studies have demonstrated the chemical alteration in the brain produced by exposure to MSG. The message here is, if there is any risk for cancer or if cancer is present, stay away from these free-radical and lipid-peroxidation promoters.

Naturally, the food industry attempts to spin the reality of toxicity by reminding us that glutamate is a naturally occurring amino acid found in many foods. The answer here, of course, is that when glutamate is free and unbound, it can be as toxic as MSG. Hydrolyzed vegetable protein is a common food additive and contains glutamate and cysteic acid, both of which are excitotoxins producing the same brain lesions as MSG or aspartame. Homocysteine is also an excitotoxin and is shown to be a major risk factor for cardiovascular disease and strokes. Researchers for the food giants clamor on about glutamate not being able to reach an intact blood-brain barrier, but this is not true because glutamate has been shown to enter the brain when there is a chronic elevation of blood glutamate present.

Neurodegenerative diseases occur for a multitude of reasons, including:

- Alterations in glucose metabolism.

- Altered neural membranes, which make an aging brain more vulnerable to excitotoxins.

- Declining energy production (mitochondrial diseases). Mitochondria—the powerhouses of the cells—provide energy to the cells in the form of ATP (the cells' primary energy source) to carry out cellular functions. Any weakness in this process can damage or destroy the mitochondria, thereby causing problems in the cells and cellular death.

- Excitotoxity.

- Free-radical generation.

- Impaired flood flow.

- Lipid peroxidation (the breakdown process for fat).

Combinations of nutrients and supplements can reduce excitotoxicity, particularly acetyl-L-carnitine, coenzyme Q_{10}, methylcobalamin, niacinamide, and phosphatidylserine.

Of special concern is the consumption of aspartame and MSG-containing products by pregnant women during the brain-formation phase of the fetus because these excitotoxins have a negative effect on the development of the baby's nervous system. For you, as the consumer, it is important to know which foods contain MSG (monosodium glutamate). You should know if there are hidden ways the food processors are including MSG (or free glutamate) in the food, without being required to put monosodium glutamate in the list of ingredients on the label. Here is a list of ingredients to be on the lookout for:

- Anything fermented, protein-fortified, or ultra-pasteurized

- Autolyzed yeast

- Barley malt, broth, or boullion

- Calcium caseinate

- Carrageen natural flavoring, gelatin

- Hydrolyzed oat flour

- Hydrolyzed protein, malt extract

- Hydrolyzed vegetable

- Natural flavors, pectin

- Plant protein extract

- Potassium glutamate

- Sodium caseinate

- Soy protein, soy sauce

- Stock textured protein

- Whey protein

- Yeast extract, yeast food

My advice is to be informed. Read labels carefully and slowly.

The average person consumes about two pounds of MSG per year. Some restaurants claim they do not use MSG in their food. Chinese restaurants use soy sauce in their cooking, and it does have MSG in it. Monosodium glutamate intensifies flavor and is now used more than ever for this purpose in fish, frozen products, hot dogs, poultry, salad dressings, sauces, and soups. It is also used as a blending agent for mixed spices. Low-fat, low-salt, low-sugar foods are all doctored for good taste, and MSG salt has actually replaced the low-sodium chloride. But what is great for the food processors is not good for the consumer.

Some individuals can tolerate MSG, but many cannot. As per my wife's experience, the reaction to MSG can be sudden, or it can take twenty-four hours. MSG is used in university research labs to enhance the laboratory animals' weight (some labs encourage animals to gain weight). What do you think MSG is doing for you?

Obesity can occur without increasing your food intake. Hunger and cravings for more is part of the MSG plan. And *No MSG* on the label is still not your security blanket because free glutamates can have the same effects. Some symptoms of both MSG and glutamate consumption include bronchospasms, a burning sensation in the face, neck, arms, and chest, chest pains, drowsiness, headaches, nausea, rapid pulse, tingling of extremities, and weakness.

The information here helps make you an informed consumer, so the next step is to prepare your own foods from fresh sources as much as possible. When you eat out, be particular about what you order and communicate your concerns to the server. Tell that person you are a 911 for MSG and could become really ill if the food contains this or any unnatural sweeteners. The server and the chef should be responsive.

Why doesn't your general practitioner or internist warn you of these dangers? Partly because of the rush-'em-through nature of HMOs, a subject of numerous articles and books, and partly because these perils haven't filtered down from neuroscientists and surgeons to the general medical community.

YOUR BRAIN HEALTH PLAN

You may feel slightly beleaguered by all this bad news, but the good news is that there is much you can do to keep your brain working at peak performance. The focus of *The Brainpower Plan* is to educate you on facts versus myths, and to get you to take an active role into your brain health, so that you can be an informed consumer.

You can do this, I know, because the one word that I use above all to describe the human brain is *flexible*. Unlike other organs, which are more or less fixed in function, the brain isn't rigid, it's a living, malleable organ affected by daily stress, diets, environments, frequency of exercise, and all the other factors that influence this amazing organ.

As with any life-changing process, brain health is all about self-empowerment. Once you recognize the importance of the diet/brain health connection, you are on a path to setting the foundation for your longevity.

I will provide a list of dietary friends and foes as the basis for a nutritional plan to help you optimize your brain health. First I would like to establish a strategy to help keep your brain in prime condition by helping you understand why this plan is vital to your life. Here are some highlights:

- Balance your glucose (sugar) to enhance production of your energy for movement.

- Eliminate toxic foods and chemical additives from your diet.

- Include amino acids in your diet. They form proteins vital to the production of neurotransmitters, which allow the brain cells to communicate.

- Include fruits and vegetables for their nutrients, which protect the cells from deterioration and dysfunction.

- Supplement your diet by adding omega-3 fatty acids, which protect cells.

HOW NUTRITION IMPACTS BRAIN HEALTH

The brain is governed by neuromodulators—brain chemicals that foster or inhibit the transmission of nerve impulses. The brain must maintain optimal flexibility to keep its thinking ability acute, so it is necessary to give the brain whatever it requires through a superior diet, exercise, and supplements.

The most common causes of brain deterioration are both the lack of nutrient-rich foods in the diet and vitamin/mineral deficiencies, which strongly contribute to the loss of memory as you age. Although manufacturers present their products as being nutritionally sufficient, a daily commercial multivitamin, such as One-A-Day, is absolutely *not* sufficient to cure functional brain problems or prevent brain disease. In truth, there is no replacement for an optimal diet of nutrient-rich foods and not even the costliest multivitamins guarantee absorption as you grow older. The need for supplementation is driven by the toxicity of the foods you ingest, as well as by the quality of those foods. Nothing could counteract the harmful effects of additives in the processed foods that most North Americans ingest on a daily basis. The only way is to take action and stop eating processed foods.

By reading labels and avoiding the main culprits among food additives and chemical preparations in processed foods, you *will* augment your brain function. A concerted effort to add brainpower super heroes to your daily diet will ensure that you avoid the painful loss of cognition and memory and have a lifetime of good brain health.

NOURISHING YOUR BRAIN

The bottom line is that optimum nutrition creates a beneficial biochemical environment to help the body boost its immune system and prevent the onset of degenerative diseases. This is true of the internal organs, and most critically true for the brain. Creating this biochemical environment in your daily life improves:

- Awareness and focus.
- Cognitive ability.
- Concentration.
- Energy levels.
- The way you feel.

Your metabolism is a key player. Metabolism refers to the chemical changes that occur in living cells, and it helps provide energy for the vital processes and activities of a given set of cells. In large part, metabolic pathways are created by what you ingest—the good, the bad, and the ugly. After eating, food is broken down into molecules, then absorbed and distributed throughout the body. Thus, how the brain is fed has a very direct impact on the health and quality of life. Brain foods set the stage for living and brain longevity. Maintaining a nutrient-rich diet free of excitotoxins and other harmful additives will keep your brain functioning at its peak level.

FIVE SUPER STRATEGIES FOR BRAIN HEALTH

STRATEGY 1—AVOID FOODS CONTAINING EXCITOTOXINS

As discussed earlier in the chapter, much of the food consumed by the average American is loaded with additives that have proven to produce serious health problems in the brain and beyond. The most pernicious of these are excitotoxins, the man-made chemicals that first appeared in the food supply in the 1940's to enhance the taste of foods. Americans eat more excitotoxins, found everywhere in frozen and packed foods, than people in France, Italy, or Spain. In fact, the food supply in developing countries is many times safer than America's. These chemicals are particularly harmful to people who have a history of various diseases. Food additives in the diet are among the most damaging health concerns of all.

✗ Aspartame

The most commonly used artificial sweetener in North America is also the most deadly excitotoxin in widespread use. This substance, the basis of such sugar substitutes as NutraSweet, is found in untold numbers of desserts, diet foods, and low-calorie sodas. The prevalence of these products in grocery stores or in your pantry makes them especially insidious foods.

Aspartic acid is an amino acid found normally in the body. Its transmission is required for us to function as healthy, fully developed individuals. When heavy doses of this artificially manufactured aspartic acid in aspartame, and its chemical cousin glutamate, react with neuronal receptors in the brain and spinal cord, it eventually results in injury and death. As a consequence, the overabundance of these acids has been irrevocably linked to neurodegenera-

The Bressler Report

Jerome Bressler was the team leader at GD Searle Company, which was attempting to gain FDA approval for aspartame as a food additive. He identified many of the deficiencies in the tests that were performed, and his report was such a damning document about aspartame that the company was obliged to conduct bogus tests with lab animals. When the lab tests indicated that rats had brain tumors and atrophied testicles, as well as other anomalies, there was obvious concern. The increase in brain tumors in the experimental animals exposed to aspartame was dose-related—the higher the dose, the higher the incidence of brain tumors. There was a forty-sevenfold increase in brain tumors in the mice, and the longer they were exposed to aspartame, the higher their incidence of tumors; the older mice were particularly susceptible to developing tumors.

Using the Freedom of Information Act, Barbara Mullarky supplied this report to the public. It is available in its entirety from the Monsanto Corporation, which purchased the GD Searle Company and which is the main manufacturer of NutraSweet. An authority on aspartame's effect on human health, H.J. Roberts, M.D., who wrote *Aspartame (NutraSweet), Is It Safe?* discussed the myth of "the most thoroughly tested additive in history." These writings and the many published studies on aspartame all demonstrate the shortcomings of the substance, yet this neurotoxin is still approved and being marketed for human consumption.

tive diseases and the brain-fog syndrome. This memory loss and intellectual deterioration can begin to appear in late middle age.

There is sufficient medical literature available to document the damage and injuries caused by food additives. More than 200 million Americans consume artificial sweeteners containing aspartame, and more than 4,000 products on the market contain this excitotoxin.. When you add up the harmful effects of ingesting aspartame, MSG, and other excitotoxins, the cumulative effect destroys the brain cells. This leads to degenerative diseases of the brain.

✗ Monosodium Glutamate (MSG)

How did MSG enter our collective consciousness in the first place? Early in the last century, chemists discovered a taste-enhancing ingredient from a Japanese seaweed called kombu or sea tangle. This naturally occurring chemical, monosodium glutamate, augments the flavor of many types of food. After World War II, millions of pounds of it were produced by laboratories around the world, forming the basis of a multimillion dollar industry. A Japanese company, Ajinomoto, is the leading producer of MSG. They also manufacture another very harmful excitotoxin, hydrolyzed vegetable protein.

In its natural form, MSG is an amino acid derived from the enzyme and hormonal system of a living plant. Initially, MSG, both natural and manmade, was thought to be safe. However, by the late 1960s, research data began indicating that MSG could have extremely deleterious effects on human health. John W. Olney, M.D., a neuroscientist at Washington University, discovered that critical parts of mice brains, and the hypothalamus (crucial to overall brain function), were destroyed after receiving only a single dose of MSG. Dr. Olney was especially concerned about the increasing use of MSG in baby foods consumed by millions of infants across the globe. His laboratory research showed beyond all doubt that young test animals were far more vulnerable to the effects of MSG than adult animals.

The FDA, however, refused to take action, and food manufacturers refused to remove MSG from their products despite the presence of irrefutable scientific evidence from a major American medical school. Undaunted, Dr. Olney persevered, eventually testifying before a congressional committee, and after years and great personal expense, Dr. Olney accomplished his mission when Congress mandated that MSG be removed from all baby foods. Most emergency room physicians have had experience diagnosing and treating the ravages of an MSG attack.

Your Anti-Excitotoxin Food Strategy

1. Look for fresh produce at organic markets.

2. Buy your spices in a spice store or gourmet shop.

3. Read labels to look for any excitotoxins.

4. Use fresh ingredients to flavor your food.

Three cheers for the fact that spices are the new heroes of modern gastronomy, especially in these health-conscious times. In fact, if you follow food trends, you will know that even old-line French chefs are extolling the virtues of fresh spices over sauces and creams. I am pleased to see metropolitan areas and smaller cities boasting spice shops. Change your *fast taste* habit with fresh-ground spices or herbs. I promise: You will cultivate a taste for fresh seasonings. Buy an organically fed bird and use any of the following: basil, cilantro, rosemary, or even ginger, and you will be quite pleased. Seasoned salt is an excitotoxin, but sea salt and kosher salt are safe.

An informed consumer is a smart shopper, and more importantly, a healthy one. I strongly suggest you read, *Excitotoxins: The Taste That Kills,* by neurosurgeon Russell Blaylock. This book provides extensive, and compelling, scientific documentation on the role of excitotoxins in the destruction of human memory, as well as their relationship to chronic neurodegenerative diseases, such as Alzheimer's and Parkinson's.

Your Anti-Excitotoxin Supplement Strategy

Chapter 7 contains a full list of brain-health supplements, but here are some specifically geared to counterbalance the collective effects of excitotoxins you have eaten in your lifetime. I recommend that all adults take the following supplements daily, in addition to your daily multivitamin/mineral capsule:

- Acetyl-L-carnitine, 1,000 mg a day

- Alpha-lipoic acid, 300 mg twice a day

- ATP, 20 mg a day, sublingually

- Idebenone, 45 mg twice a day

- Magnesium, 300 mg a day

- NADH, 5 mg a day on an empty stomach

- Selenium, 200 mg a day

- Vitamin C, 1,000 mg, three times a day

- Vitamin E (mixed tocopherols), 400 mg a day

- Zinc, 15 mg a day

STRATEGY 2—EAT FOODS RICH IN ANTIOXIDANTS

Although essential for life, oxygen does create damaging body products known as free radicals, which are analogous to rust collecting on unprotected iron, cut apples turning brown, or butter turning rancid. Free radicals are also created by exposure to toxins—tobacco smoke and radiation. If uncontrolled, these free radicals damage cell walls, cell structure, and genetic material within the cells. Antioxidants protect the cell components by neutralizing these free radicals, but as their defense is not 100 percent effective, damaged cells can still accumulate and contribute to neurodegenerative diseases, such as Alzheimer's and Parkinson's.

A recent study by the American Heart Association Scientific Session showed that women who consumed higher amounts of antioxidant-containing foods had a 33 percent lower risk of a heart attack and a startling 71 percent lower risk of a stroke than women who ate few antioxidant-containing foods. The American Academy in Nutritional Research (AANR) has suggested that antioxidants slow the progress, and even reverse the propensity, for heart disease and strokes. It has been shown that antioxidants can influence cholesterol in the bloodstream by increasing levels of HDL (good) cholesterol and reducing LDL (bad) cholesterol.

Foods rich in antioxidants include broccoli, cabbage, carrots, kale, red and green peppers, spinach, squash, tomatoes, and yams. But whether the antioxidants are taken in the form of food or supplements, they protect the cells and their components by neutralizing free radicals, in medical terms, quenching the radicals. You should do everything in your power to increase the antioxidants in your body. I urge you to think about this commitment as one of the most effective you can make to achieve a long life of excellent health and to avoid many progressive brain diseases.

The research of Jeffrey Hampl, Ph.D., R.D., at Arizona University, reaffirms the fact that it is vital for people to increase their consumption of foods rich in vitamin C, which is the strongest antioxidant available by diet. "Low intake of vegetables and fruits, especially citrus fruits, leads to inadequate vitamin-C intake among adults." Previous research revealed that only 20 percent of adults consume the recommended five daily servings of fruits and vegetables. However, there is concern that some of the adults consuming the five servings of fruits and vegetables are still deficient in vitamin C (humans and other primates are the only animal species that cannot synthesize vitamin C, but must get it from food or supplements).

The latest government recommendation for vitamin C for adults is 60 mg per day, which is a laughably insufficient guideline to anyone familiar with alternative health standards. A study showed that 42 percent of American adults who are not taking adequate vitamin-C supplements needed to include more foods containing vitamin C in their diet. The list of the important functions of vitamin C (ascorbic acid) is vast, and includes, besides its original use to prevent scurvy, its ability to improve the integrity of blood vessels.

The August 1996 issue of *The American Journal of Clinical Nutrition* published the results of a compelling study showing that a high-potency antioxidant supplement, such as vitamin E, can reduce atherosclerosis (hardening of the arteries). This nine-year study from 1984 to 1993 involved 11,178 older people, who participated in the trial to establish the effects of vitamin supplements on mortality. The results showed that vitamin E reduced the risk of death from all causes by 34 percent, and the effects were strongest for coronary artery disease, where the use of vitamin E resulted in a 63 percent reduction in death from heart attacks and strokes. In addition, the use of vitamin E resulted in a 59 percent reduction in cancer mortality. When the effects of vitamin C and E were compared, overall mortality was reduced by 42 percent (compared to 34 percent for vitamin E alone). At this time, many trials are being conducted to determine the effectiveness of vitamin E in protecting against dementia or cognitive decline.

The Antioxidant Food Plan

There are three major groups of antioxidant foods. Here I provide a list of the key antioxidants in each category, along with serving sizes, as recommended by the USDA. The way to use this guide is to choose at least one helping from each of the three groups to get the minimum daily requirements of antioxidants to help ensure brain health. Unlike animal protein, and excepting the vegetable oil, you can't eat too many of these brain foods.

The food sources for antioxidants are numerous, and include:

- Fruits, including cantaloupes, grapefruit, kiwi, oranges, peaches, and strawberries
- Nuts, seeds, and wheat germ
- Seafood

Foods rich in vitamin C include:

- Asparagus, 1 cup
- Broccoli, cooked, ½ cup
- Brussels sprouts, fresh, 1 cup
- Cantaloupe, ½ cup
- Cranberry juice, ¾ cup
- Kiwi, 1 fruit
- Orange juice, ¾ cup
- Orange, 1 fruit
- Papaya, 1 cup
- Potato, baked, 1 medium
- Red pepper, ¼ cup
- Spinach, 1 cup
- Strawberries, fresh, ½ cup
- Vegetable juice, ½ cup

Foods rich in vitamin E include:

- Grains (organically grown grain cereals, oat and rice bran)
- Nuts and seeds. (Almonds, hazelnuts [filberts], sunflower seeds), ⅓ cup each
- Spinach, ½ cup
- Sweet potato, 1 medium
- Wheat germ, toasted, ¼ cup

- Vegetable oils, canola, olive, sunflower, counted as part of your vitamin E

Research involving carotenoids (yellow to red pigments) found them to be valuable antioxidants abundant in fruits and vegetables that help preserve brain function into old age. Dutch researchers in this Rotterdam Study concluded that carotenoid intake lessened lesions in the white matter of the brain that were located adjacent to the ventricles containing the cerebrospinal fluid. This suggests that these potent antioxidants may slow the development of atherosclerosis by inhibiting the oxidation of low-density lipoprotein (LDL) within the arterial wall.

In addition, carotenoids may help preserve the integrity of brain tissue by scavenging free-radical oxygen molecules that, if left unopposed, can cause cellular damage. Brain lesions develop over a period of time, which necessitates a long-term commitment to good nutrition (people who eat plenty of fruits and vegetables are also more likely to exercise regularly and not smoke).

Foods rich in carotenoids include:

- Butternut squash, ½ cup
- Cantaloupe, ½ cup
- Carrot, ½ cup
- Collard greens, 1 cup
- Kale, 1 cup
- Mango, ½ cup
- Mustard greens, ½ cup
- Peas and carrots, ½ cup
- Pumpkin, ½ cup
- Sweet potato, 1 medium
- Swiss chard, ½ cup
- Vegetable juice, ¾ cup
- Vegetables, mixed, ½ cup

Note: All fruits and vegetables should be fresh; amounts given are for whole fruit and cooked vegetables.

STRATEGY 3—AVOID A DIET PROMOTING EXCESS PRODUCTION OF INSULIN

Until recently, most people did not think twice about insulin. It was thought to be related only to diabetes, and not as something for anyone in good health to be concerned about. However, with the popularity of such diet books as *Enter the Zone* and *Sugar Busters!,* the subject of blood sugar has crept to the forefront of health consciousness. And with good reason: Our awareness of insulin levels is crucial to maintaining optimal body weight, but insulin also plays a major role in our long-term brain health (*see* Chapter 9).

What is insulin? It is a hormone essential for the conversion of carbohydrates into energy and is therefore integral to human health. In excess, however, insulin can severely damage cells, especially the brain cells crucial to cognitive ability, memory, and long-term health. In addition, excess insulin affects aging negatively by causing both nerve and brain-cell degeneration.

For these reasons, managing insulin levels remains a high priority for brain health. To manage it properly, it is necessary to know the glycemic index levels of different foods. This index was originally established for people with diabetes, but it has turned into a standard measure to determine the risk of elevated blood sugar that occurs with certain carbohydrates, and it is considered an important information resource about carbohydrate ingestion.

Dr. David Jenkins, a nutrition professor at the University of Toronto, led researchers to classify foods according to their glycemic index, which refers to the immediate rise in blood sugar that occurs following the ingestion of foods containing carbohydrates.

- **High-glycemic-index foods.** The rapid digestion of foods, including refined carbohydrates, will lead to a fast release of glucose in the bloodstream.

- **Low-glycemic-index foods.** The slow digestion of foods, including complex carbohydrates, will lead to a slow release of glucose into the bloodstream.

How Scientists Measure the Glycemic Index

The glycemic index list assigns a numerical value to food. A standard amount of carbohydrates (25–50 grams) are given to a volunteer to eat. Over the next two hours, a blood sample is taken every fifteen minutes for one hour, and thereafter every thirty minutes for an additional hour or two. These blood-glucose levels are measured and recorded, then the numbers are compared with the blood-glucose response to 50 grams of pure glucose, known as the reference food, which is tested on two or three separate occasions. The average glycemic index value found in eight to ten people gives the value (number) of that food.

Why is this index important? By experiencing a gradual rise and fall in the blood-glucose response, the test subjects are controlling the insulin secretion. Slow digestion helps to minimize hunger pains and promote weight loss in obese people. There are fewer glycemic spikes so coronary health can be improved by the reduction of oxidative stress. These spikes are related to the necessary insulin response. Insulin exerts an anti-cell-death activity by suppressing the excessive accumulation of reactive oxygen species (free radical production). This control of the blood-glucose levels ensures that the blood vessels remain elastic, and this can help reduce arteriosclerosis and lower any tendency to form blood clots, which place the brain or heart in jeopardy.

History is a base to learn from, and in this instance it describes nutrition of the past, meaning slow-released foods, which did not then incur the wrath of insulin. Originally whole and natural complex-carbohydrate foods were remade into fast-release or refined *insulin food* as part of a convenient food supply whose main concern is a longer shelf life. These foods did not retain the rich nutrients needed for your brain. And the result of this is now catching up with people via such conditions as heart disease, obesity, strokes, and type II diabetes. The glycemic index is only a guideline of information for you to make proper choices related to carbohydrate and sugar-rich foods. The benefits of different foods are varied, and you should make food choices based on the nutritional content of the food—fiber, salt, saturated fat, and now the glycemic index, as a guide to carbohydrate intake.

The Glycemic Index—A Guide to Carbohydrate Intake

Insulin is a *storage* hormone involved in glucose, protein, and fat. The idea that food and a low-glycemic index have an effect on fat loss is based on the conclusion that these foods help control insulin levels. Here are a few facts concerning insulin:

- Insulin increases the fat-storage enzyme, lipoprotein lipase (LPL), which promotes the storage of fat.

- Insulin inhibits lipase, an enzyme responsible for breaking down stored fat.

- Insulin activates the enzyme acetyl coenzyme A-carboxylase, which, along with the fatty acid synthase, is utilized to convert carbohydrates into fat.

TABLE 6.1. THE GLYCEMIC INDEX FOR COMMON FOODS

The numbers next to the food indicate the actual glycemic value, with sugar (glucose) being at 100.

Low GI Food—below 55 • Intermediate GI Food—55 to 70
High GI Food—more than 70

Intermediate to High GI		Low GI	
Fruits			
Cantaloupe	65	Apples	30
Papaya	56	Grapes	45
Pineapple	65	Kiwi fruit	50
Watermelon	70	Oranges	50
		Peaches	40
		Plums	25
Starchy Foods			
Corn, sweet	60	Beans, baked	38
French fries	75	Beans, lentils	46
Potato, baked	82	Pasta, capellini	45
Potato, boiled	82	Pasta, vermicelli	35
Potato, mashed	82	Potato, sweet	44
Rice cakes	80	Rice, basmati	38
Rice, converted Uncle Ben's	58	Rice noodles	40
Rice, instant	90		
Bread Products			
Bagels	75	Sourdough bread	48
French bread	95	Wholegrain bread	51
Hamburger buns	90		
Rolls, white	90		
Scones	92		
White bread	90		
Whole wheat bread	65		

Intermediate to High GI		Low GI	
Cereals			
Cocoa Puffs	77	All-Bran	30
Corn Flakes	92	Frosted Flakes	55
Fruit Loops	69	Muesli	43
Rice Krispies	82	Oatmeal, old-fashioned	55
		Special K	55
Cookies			
Sugar wafer w/filling	77	Social Tea Biscuits	45
Oreo, reduced fat	67	Oatmeal	55
Snacks			
Fruit bars	61	Almonds	0
Ice cream, chocolate	68	Apricots, dried	30
Ice cream, vanilla	50	Brazil nuts	0
Popcorn	72	Cherries, dried	40
Pretzels	83	Dates	50
		Peanuts	14
		Prunes	29
		Yogurt, low-fat	31

Source: Dr. Simin Liu, Harvard University School of Public Health
This data represents the findings of the Harvard Nurses Health Study

TABLE 6.2. TOP TWENTY SOURCES OF CARBOHYDRATES—STANDARD AMERICAN DIET

1. Potatoes, baked or mashed	6. Bananas	11. Fruit punch	16. White sugar
2. White bread	7. White rice	12. Coca-Cola	17. Jam
3. Cold cereal	8. Pizza	13. Apples	18. Cranberry juice
4. Dark bread	9. Pasta	14. Skim milk	19. French fries
5. Orange juice	10. Muffins	15. Pancakes	20. Candy

Source: Dr. Simin Liu, Harvard University School of Public Health
This data represents the findings of the Harvard Nurses Health Study

From this discussion, you can see that high levels of insulin make it less likely for the fat already stored around your middle to be converted into energy.

You choose how much carbohydrate you eat, but be aware that the type of carbohydrate (and fat) you choose is important, as is the amount you consume—one size does not fit all. Balance is the answer, and if you feel it is necessary, you can consult a nutrition expert, at least at the beginning. If you don't know a nutrition expert, you can contact your local hospital or the American Dietetic Association (*see* Resources in back).

STRATEGY 4—EAT FEWER ANIMAL PROTEINS

Forget the Mercedes. It's red meat that is the universal marker of status and wealth. In Japan, Kobe beef is expensive and prized. In northern Italy, a huge Florentine steak is a symbol of wealth, and in America and Canada, people without financial concerns may remember their parents' serving them meat at most dinners. Red meat and poultry are undoubtedly good sources of protein, and they also supply essential B vitamins, iron, and zinc. But human beings need far less protein to thrive than is commonly assumed. An active person weighing 150 pounds needs only 75–115 grams of protein per day. The brainpower food plan presented here will give you a good idea of just how much of each food you need in your daily diet. For now, know that you can get all the protein your brain and body need by eating the following every day:

- Two 8-ounce servings low-fat milk (20 grams); or

- 3 ounces of turkey in a sandwich (25 grams); or

- A handful of peanuts for a midday snack (25 grams); or

- 4 ounces of red meat at dinner (30 grams).

Even if you are closer to 200 pounds and exceptionally active, you would only need several extra ounces of protein a day to fill your daily requirement of protein. Your body just can't use or process more protein than this.

There is a far more salient reason to limit your intake than mere calorie counting. The saturated fats that all animal meats contain are a recognized marker for heart disease and strokes. Also, an excess of protein can cause disorders of the liver and kidney. In fact, in the last fifty years, the overabundance of animal protein in the diet—in most industrialized countries, people eat two to three times as much protein as the body requires—has been a major contributing factor to increasing maladies.

If the health connection doesn't spur you into action, maybe the weight connection will. Excess protein is converted into carbohydrates and stored by the body as fat, and, as of now, obesity is epidemic. More than 54 percent of Americans are overweight, and this condition affects not only their stamina and physical appearance, but is a known precursor to neurological dysfunction that includes hypertension and strokes.

As if this weren't bad enough, there is another very compelling reason to limit intake of excess animal protein. This excess protein is associated with kidney stones and osteoporosis, as well as some cancers. If you are a heavy meat eater, you are vulnerable for all these conditions, but by restricting your diet, as much as possible, to low-fat meats, you may avoid these diseases. Your best bets are lean beef, pork, or veal; bison; ostrich; skinless free-range chicken; turkey; and venison.

The National Academy of Science's Food and Nutrition Board advises that 0.57 grams of protein for every kilogram (2.2 pounds) of body weight is sufficient and can be achieved by eating plant protein, rather than animal protein. You need not avoid animal protein entirely if you make smart choices and choose lean cuts. Even hamburger, that most vilified of food stuffs, can be occasionally enjoyed if you buy lean or extra-lean ground beef.

Preparation Tips

Use a paper towel or an extra bun to drain the grease from your burger. If you are making spaghetti sauce with ground beef, pork, or veal, remember to absorb the fat with paper towels or use a colander after cooking but before adding them to the sauce. While the meat is still in the colander, rinse it with hot water to remove even more fat. This method lets you have your meat and eat it too. When you order a hamburger in a restaurant, ask for an extra bun, which will absorb the grease.

Dangers do occur from preparing meat and poultry, so it is important to:

- Clean the food (this is absolutely essential).

- Rinse the poultry before cooking.

- Refrigerate meat and poultry while marinating.

- Cook beef until it is medium pink (160°F).

- Cook pork until it is just pink (160°F).

Beneficial Protein Sources

Active people who eat a lot of meat may consume too few carbohydrates, which can cause fatigue (carbohydrates replace the glycogen that the muscles use up). The recommended 3–4-ounce portion of meat provides adequate protein. Remember to eat small portions of the leanest cuts. It is not responsible to recommend a high-protein, high-fat diet, which results in much higher levels of chronic degenerative diseases.

Vegetable proteins are as equally effective and nutritious as meat proteins—soybeans have twice the amount of protein found in meat (soybeans contain 41 percent protein and lean-cut beefsteak contains 20 percent protein). Recent studies have again shown that animal proteins increase cholesterol, and plant proteins tend to reduce cholesterol in both animals and humans. Among the best sources of vegetable-based protein to include in your diet are:

- Beans (legumes), lentils, and tofu
- Fresh vegetables, such as baby bok choy, and zucchini

The basis of the vegetarian approach to diet is the ability to obtain the vital protection needed from plants and fruits, but unless you are philosophically or morally committed to vegetarianism, there is no reason to give up animal protein entirely. A much better plan of action is to gradually ease vegetable sources into your diet. Choose a falafel sandwich for lunch instead of a turkey burger. There are many creative food exchanges. It will benefit your brain *and* your digestive system when you choose to make them.

The popular belief that fruits and vegetables have the greatest risk of pesticide contamination has been recently refuted by FDA studies. In fact, domestic fish products contain more pesticide residues than fruits, grains, or vegetables. Freshwater fish, such as trout caught in inland lakes, are the most vulnerable to contamination by dioxin carcinogens, and, as of now, coldwater fish from deep in the sea are found to have the least contamination.

The major benefit of fish consumption is its omega-3 fatty-acid content, which has a positive effect on the blood vessels, heart, and rheumatoid arthritis. Omega-3 fatty acids can also be obtained from plant sources, such as canola oil, flaxseed oil, and walnuts.

STRATEGY 5—AVOID TRANS-FATTY ACIDS AND HYDROGENATED OILS

Newspaper columnist David Lawrence Dewey was right on target when he told us that the American diet contains "10–44 percent of trans-fatty acids in commercially prepared foods and they are deadly to the human body." Frank Sachs, M.D., on the faculty of the Harvard School of Public Health, wrote in *The New England Journal of Medicine:* "American food manufacturers are manipulating our foods in a way that refutes scientific research and shows that trans-fatty acids compromise health. Furthermore, the lack of information on trans-fatty acids on food labels does not allow one to make an informed decision or choice."

What are trans-fatty acids and hydrogenated oils? Neither occurs in nature; they are, instead, man-made compounds that have been artificially formulated to prolong the shelf life of many commercially available foods. Because these acid molecular structures have been altered, the human body does not recognize them, which means they cannot transport vital minerals and other nutrients to our cell membranes.

At best, when eating foods containing hydrogenated oils, you are eating empty calories. But the situation is actually much worse than that because these oils have been manufactured by hydrogenated gas via metal catalysts, including aluminum, cobalt, and nickel. Because these metals are toxic to the human body, eating foods manufactured with hydrogenated or partially hydrogenated oils can have devastating health effects. By lingering in the body, they promote a deterioration of the fatty part of the brain. This fragile breakdown of brain function eventually results in diseases that include Alzheimer's, Parkinson's, and strokes.

Trans-fatty acids also take a potentially deadly toll on the human body by:

- Causing a low birth weight when consumed by pregnant women.

- Causing breast cancer.

- Decreasing testosterone levels, causing aberrations of sperm.

- Elevating cholesterol levels by as much as 30 percent.

- Heightening the risk of heart disease.

- Increasing free-radical formation (remember the peeled apple).

Alarmist? No, not if you believe the Harvard researchers, or me, or the decision made by Denmark. This Scandinavian country, whose concern for its citizenry is unrivaled among nations, has banned the commercial use of hydrogenated oils for more than forty years. It is no coincidence, I believe, that the land of the Danes has the lowest rates of breast cancer, diabetes, heart disease, and diseases of the immune system in the world. Unlike Denmark, where the citizenry's health and welfare is the government's primary concern, the United States often puts big business first and shelf life becomes more important than your life.

Some of my patients believe these chemically altered hydrogenated oils are only found in products they don't eat, but they need to think again. Among the more commonly consumed food items that contain hydrogenated oils and other trans-fatty acids are cookies, crackers, potato chips, even frozen quiche. And margarine, once touted as healthy, is composed of nothing but potentially deadly hydrogenated oils.

There are trans-fatty acids in many packaged frozen foods, but they pale in comparison to the amount found in nearly all fast foods. McDonald's announced they were changing from a trans-fatty oil for French fries, but this was put on hold, and a large order of fries still has 540 calories. They have, under consumer pressure, managed to reduce the amount of fat in their French fries, but they are still laden with trans-fatty acids, as are the fries you buy at Arby's or Hardee's. There are more trans-fatty acids in the fries at Burger King or Wendy's than at any other chain.

Fresh fish from uncontaminated waters is healthy, but that is not the case for most fish and chips restaurants, and certainly not for Red Lobster's "Admirals Feast," a menu selection that could cause brain damage in a whole boatload of sailors. But even this fat-laden food is a walk in the nutritional park compared to a typical Kentucky Fried Chicken meal. You can eat a five-piecer with fries if you must, but buy a good life insurance policy beforehand.

Finally, as if there weren't enough reasons not to eat Dunkin' (or any other) doughnuts, the treasure trove of traps they contain—fatty acids—is another good one. In addition to the risk of brain damage these fatty acids can cause, there is the threat of high cholesterol and heart disease. Eating just one Dunkin' Donut is equivalent to *eight* strips of bacon.

In the United States, the amount of unhealthy trans fats hidden in such foods as margarine and Oreo cookies is no longer a secret. For years nothing was done about their adverse effects because of opposition from the food industry. In early July 2003, however, in the first major labeling change since 1993, the FDA announced that, effective January 2006, there will be new food labeling which will require manufacturers to list, under the saturated fats on the label, any trans-fatty acids in the product. In this way, it will be easy to add up the two types of harmful fats and get the *true* number for blood-vessel damage. The foot-dragging FDA was pushed to act by the science presented to it. To his credit, FDA commissioner Mark B. McClellan said, "Our choices about our diets are choices about our health, and those choices should be based on the best scientific information. This label change means that trans fat can no longer lurk, hidden, in our food choices." Good for Mark.

Here's a surprise for you. According to the label, a doughnut contains 5 grams of saturated fat, but trans fats not yet listed on the label add *another* 5 grams to the bad fats, for 10 grams total. Margo G. Wootan, the director of the Nutrition Policy Center for Science in the Public Interest said, "That is half a day's worth of artery-clogging fat in one doughnut—nobody can fit that into a healthy diet." Both saturated fat and trans fat together should provide *less* than 8 to 10 percent of the daily calories, about 20 grams of fat.

The message has been delivered to the manufacturers and it may spur them to remove the trans-fats from processed foods—chips, cookies, margarine, etc.—before 2006. A few companies are taking these much needed steps, since trans-fats lower the HDL (good) cholesterol, and this is in addition to all the other damage they do. The Bestfoods company was scheduled to remove trans fats from their I Can't Believe It's Not Butter spreads in mid 2004. Frito-Lay has plans to introduce fat-free Cheetos, Doritos, and Tostitos, and Kraft has said they will start to trim the trans fats from their products. In the meantime, however, how many avoidable coronary occlusions and strokes will occur from all the other processed foods filling every supermarket shelf in the country?

Healthy Fats

The concern about too much fat in our diets is warranted, but it is also important to have sufficient amounts of the beneficial high-quality oils that can be vital for health. Fats are critical in the creation of each cell; they are the building blocks of hormones and are vital in the development of the nervous system—and the highly processed oils undergoing hydrogenation reduce many of the healthy components of these good oils.

- **Monounsaturated fats** help to relax muscles affected by saturated fats. The leading distributor of healthy oils, Spectrum Naturals, states that almond, avocado, olive, canola, peanut, safflower, sesame, and sunflower oils have more than 50 percent monounsaturated fats.

- **Polyunsaturated fats** are composed of omega-3 and omega-6 fatty acids, and have cholesterol-lowering properties. The body cannot synthesize these oils, so you must add them to the diet. Most nutritionists say the body requires two or three times as much omega-3 as omega-6; however, in the standard American diet (SAD) the ratio is usually the reverse, and the culinary oils canola, corn, safflower, sesame, soy, and walnut are richer sources of omega-6 than omega-3. For this reason, flaxseed oil is the best vegetable source since the ratio is reversed. The latest recommendation from the American Heart Association is to use oils in equal proportion. The World Health Organization (WHO) recommends a ratio of omega-6 to omega-3 of 5 to 10 in the diet. The intake of polyunsaturated fat should be accompanied by vitamins E, C, and carotene to help prevent lipid peroxidation.

All oils require protection from heat and light so they will not oxidize and become rancid, because rancidity promotes free radicals, and even exposing oil to air increases rancidity. Frying foods speeds the process of oxidation, and oils that have been heated can be dangerous because they are carcinogenic. Omega-3 is the most sensitive oil and should be refrigerated, as should flaxseed oil, which should be used cold.

For high heat (504°F), Spectrum Naturals recommends using super canola, high-oleic safflower, peanut, soybean, or sunflower oil. For stir frying and baking (below 375°F), they recommend canola, sesame, and sunflower. For sautéing (under 320° F), they say to use olive or corn oil. The labels on Spectrum Naturals' oil products show the cooking range of each oil.

Facts about Oils

- All vegetable oils contain 100 percent fat.

- Each tablespoon of vegetable oil contains 14 grams of fat.

- Each tablespoon of vegetable oil contains 120 calories.

- For better health, choose oils or fats that are low in saturated fat.

In spite of some controversy over canola oil, it is recommended because it has low saturated-fat levels, a good balance of mono- and polyunsaturated fats, and 10 percent omega-3. Olive oil is primary in the Mediterranean diet, proving friendly to the heart and brain.

Table 6.3 shows the comparative position of saturated, polyunsaturated, and monounsaturated fats in edible vegetable oils.

TABLE 6.3. FATS AND OILS			
Type of Oil/Fat	% Saturated Fat	% Poly-unsaturated	% Mono-unsaturated
Almond Oil	8	19	73
Butter	66	4	30
Butter, whipped	69	3	28
Canola Oil	7	35	58
Cocoa Butter	62	3	35
Coconut Oil	92	2	6
Corn Oil	13	62	25
Margarine, Flora Pro-active	25	49	26
Margarine, stick	20	33	47
Margarine, tub	17	37	46
Margarine, whipped	20	30	50
Olive Oil	14	12	74
Palm Oil	52	10	38
Peanut Oil	18	33	49
Safflower Oil	9	78	13
Sesame Oil	15	43	42
Sunflower Oil	11	69	20
Walnut Oil	14	67	19
Wheatgerm Oil	20	50	30

Protect Yourself against the Effects of Hydrogenated Oils

Invest in healthy cooking for your heart and brain by reading labels on all packaged and frozen foods and use your newfound knowledge to limit your intake of processed foods, almost all of which contain trans fats. Healthy oils are sold in health food stores and in some conventional stores.

The best solution of all is to eschew processed foods; in fact, why not ban them from your diet altogether? In addition to losing weight, you will be replacing packaged products with fresh eggs, crackers with carrots, and peanut butter with fresh peanuts. You will rid your body of harmful, chemically modified oils and you will return to the diet of your ancestors who gathered and hunted, and had no concern for the silent killer, hydrogenated oil.

CHAPTER 7

Brainpower Supplements

Do or do not.
There is no try.

—YODA

I n the last chapter, I emphasized the importance of eating smart. Following a diet free of toxins will promote longevity and cognition, and by avoiding foods that can damage the brain, you will be taking important steps in securing brain health and a long, healthy life.

In an ideal world, food would be the only source needed to get all the vitamins and minerals the body required. Today, however, for the reasons discussed in this chapter, even those who take their health very seriously may lack the total nutrients required for optimal health, and supplementation—a complement of vitamins and minerals to enhance the foods eaten—becomes a must to guard against suboptimal health or disease. But, of all the subjects I cover in a patient's visit, proper supplementation is the one that causes most concern, and the one that most baffles people in general, even those who are highly educated and health conscious.

Steven, a patient with a nuclear physics degree from MIT, admitted to me that he had felt bewildered when it came to arriving at a formula for the most effective nutritional supplements. Although he recently started a supplement regimen, he said that he had taken no vitamins of any sort for years because in 1980 his internist had entirely dismissed the question of supplements. "Don't worry about vitamins," this doctor had said, "I'm sure you get enough of them from the foods you eat." This was the prevailing attitude then, when the phrase *health food* came from a few start-up stores and was not a part of the culture in the southern city where Steven grew up.

There was just one problem with the doctor's response—he hadn't even asked Steven what he ate, and if he had, he might have changed his point of view very fast. "At that time," Steven said, "I thought I ate a healthful diet if there was tomato sauce on my pepperoni pizza. In any case, it seemed a whole lot better than the fried chicken and ham hocks most people were eating."

With regard to people in the South, I interject an informational point. The southern region did offer many specialties that could only result in towering cholesterol levels. But it also is true that folks south of the Mason-Dixon Line tend to eat more farm-fresh vegetables than those in most parts of the country. This is because of the cultural eating habits in rural traditions, southern culinary affinities, and the availability of fresh produce nearly year-round.

I would like to think that Steven's story is only an interesting historical sidebar because the mainstream media is now flooded with numerous informative articles on nutrition that were formerly the stuff of alternative publications and tiny health food stores. True as that is, however, and given everything we know about nutrition today, it is still amazing how many people are nutritionally unaware, which is why I and others have chosen to educate people about improving their nutrient ingestion. Unfortunately, too many physicians have not learned of the direct link between good health and eating for a preventive lifestyle. This includes a regimen of supplementation. My patients often tell me that their doctors seem uninterested, uninformed, and dismissive about the importance of nutritional supplements for well-being and health.

And I say, "I don't care if you have to pick up her or his reflex hammer and pound it on the examination table, you have the absolute right to obtain health information about vitamin and mineral supplements as an integral part of your health profile. And if your family doctor still does not care to discuss it with you, I say find another doctor."

I realize this may be easier said than done, considering the current rush-'em-in, rush-'em-out, profit-making mentality of HMOs, but everyone is entitled to good health if they insist on it. Nowhere is the phrase *knowledge is power* more valuable than when it concerns your health.

REASONS FOR SUPPLEMENTION

Why would you require supplementation if you followed the dietary guidelines in the last chapter? Here are three valid reasons to add nutritional supplements to the diet.

1. Soil Depletion

According to the esteemed National Academy of Sciences, the average American must eat twice as many vegetables as they did twenty years ago to obtain the daily minimum requirement of most vitamins due to over-farming and the resulting depletion of minerals in the soil. It is well-established that almost all commercially grown vegetables have fewer vitamins and minerals than they had twenty years ago. For example:

- Broccoli contains less than half the vitamin A and calcium it had as recently as ten years ago.

- Cauliflower has lost half its vitamin C, thiamine, and riboflavin content.

- Pineapple, once the most calcium-rich of fruits, has lost almost all of this vital mineral.

These depressing statistics, which persist throughout the entire fruit and vegetable categories, can be laid directly at the feet of the giant agribusiness companies whose motive is profit, not health.

2. Toxic Pollution

Environmental toxins will be fully discussed in Chapter 8, but they go along with soil depletion as a reason to take supplements. This is because, in their search for profits, these giant food companies use any chemicals they deem necessary to grow more food that will ship well to market and not spoil en route. On this subject, you may have read or know about Rachel Carson's *Silent Spring,* published half a century ago. The truth she brought out is this: The earth on which we live today is vastly different from that of our forebears. Even if people were able to ingest sufficient vitamins and minerals from food sources, it would still be requisite to take supplements in order to counterbalance the extremely deleterious effects of today's highly toxic world.

3. Fragile Nutrients

This point needs emphasizing: You must be vigilant about the food you eat. You will not receive all the vitamins and minerals you think by just eating fresh fruits and vegetables because produce loses essential nutrients as quickly as six to eight hours after being picked. The very best way to ensure optimal nutrients would of course be to grow them yourself. Unless you grow your own foods organically and eat the produce soon after picking it, you cannot count on the quality of the food you buy.

Even the freshest vegetables in the best stores have already lost nutrients by the time they arrive. Worse than that, buying vegetables from a budget bin is a bad idea because that produce is only a day away from spoiling; and a low-priced store's produce is also not the freshest, that's why it's cheap. So, regardless of your economic circumstances, please don't scrimp on spending for fresh fruits or vegetables. No other food expenditure has as direct a result on the quality of your brain and overall health as the produce you eat.

Fresh is always best. Buy the best produce possible, but again, unless it's recently picked, organically grown food, buying the freshest produce still isn't any guarantee you are getting all the nutrients you need. The fungicides and other soil additives used by the giant commercial growers competes with your body by draining the soil of the vitamins and minerals you need. Again, this is one more reason why adding supplements to your diet is absolutely necessary.

FREE RADICALS AND SUPPLEMENTATION WITH ANTIOXIDANTS

Free radicals are everywhere. A natural byproduct of brain metabolism, they are dangerous molecules that result from excess oxidation. (If you visualize a cut fruit left on the kitchen counter, the browning is oxidation.) Though they are formed normally by your metabolism, these unhealthy compounds have one missing electron, and, as such, can cause major damage to tissues and cells. Most illnesses, and especially the aging process, are the result of toxic reactions formed by free radicals. What is important to understand here is that free radicals can also cause collateral damage to formerly healthy cells, which result in the progressive decline of brain function as people age.

Dr. Denham Harman formulated the free-radical theory of aging in 1967, but it took twenty-seven years, until 1994, to realize the value of his discovery. Dr. Harman implicated free radicals in fifty disorders, including Alzheimer's disease, cataracts, and rheumatoid arthritis.

Your built-in antioxidants are fighting all the time to allow you to function normally. The evidence from valid research has revealed how antioxidants are neuroprotective. Although antioxidants occur in foods, it is essential to weigh the balance in your favor and supplement with antioxidants.

The brain does not store oxygen, but constantly uses it for fuel. All brain cells require energy production from glucose and oxygen. The mitochondria (the powerhouse of the cells), is like a car engine requiring fuel, and the byproduct of the mitochondria is the production of free radicals. As people age, the mitochondria become less efficient, yet continue to produce the toxic free radicals. The destruction caused by these radicals can cross over the cell membranes, hampering protein synthesis and damaging the very mitochondria that helped to produce them, causing an early death of neurons. The interaction between free radicals and a cell membrane (which is made of fat) may cause a terminal rupture and the death of that cell. But here the plot thickens because some free radicals help kill growing cancer cells and invading bacteria, thereby giving them a beneficial role in the body.

The important point related to the brain and memory is that the hippocampal cells responsible for memory have a very high rate of oxidation and produce an enormous number of free radicals, which could be a reason for memory deterioration as people age. Stress and chronic diseases, particularly with an ineffective immune system, make the mitochondria even less efficient in countering the effects of rising oxidation. The effect on DNA within the cell nucleus may determine the extent of neurodegeneration. Aging is a free-radical disease that varies in severity. Some brains are more dysfunctional than others.

Conditions linked to free radicals include:

- Alzheimer's disease
- Arthritis
- Diabetes
- Glaucoma
- Heart disease
- Inflammatory bowel disease
- Macular degeneration
- Strokes

Outside causes of free radicals include:

- Alcohol consumption
- Buffet-style restaurants
- Chemotherapy
- Environmental pollution
- Foods that are aged or fermented (leftovers have more bacteria)
- Radiation
- Saturated and hydrogenated fats
- Smoked, cured, and barbecued meats
- Smoking and secondhand smoke
- Unusual stress

WHAT YOU CAN DO

Every outside cause of free-radical formation can be controlled to some extent, and although it's trickier inside the body, you can control production of these harmful compounds there too. The brain generates more free radicals per gram of tissue than any other organ, but you can counter this potential damage by taking supplements that protect neurons and blood vessels, thus ensuring the flow of nutrients to the brain. By following a rigorous and well-constructed plan of nutritional defense, you can do much to keep your brain healthy and prevent disease, laying the groundwork for long-term health and longevity.

Adding nutrients to your diet is your very best defense. When you get the nutrients your body needs, you are fighting the cellular degeneration that is an inevitable part of aging, at the same time that you are fighting free radicals in the most effective way.

One specific remedy includes taking more antioxidants to neutralize these destructive elements and help save your brain. Taking optimal amounts of the three main antioxidant nutrients—beta-carotene and vitamins C and E—is estimated to save 8.7 billion dollars annually by the reduction of cancer, heart disease, and strokes alone.

The Council for Responsible Nutrition (CRN), an advocate group for supplementation, estimates there would be another 20 billion annual savings for medical care and hospitalization if women of childbearing age had taken supplements.

INTRODUCTION TO VITAMINS

Vitamins (*vita* means life; *amins* denotes nitrogen compounds) were discovered close to ninety years ago. Hippocrates, the ancient Greek physician considered the father of medicine, prescribed liver for so-called night blindness (the inability to see well in dim light). The liver assists in the absorption of the fat-soluble vitamins (A, D, E, and K) because bile secretion from it converts beta-carotene into vitamin A, which helps with vision. A lack of zinc, which is needed for vitamin A to take action, can reduce vision at night. Hippocrates went to the source of where these vitamins and this mineral were stored—the liver. (Eating liver, beef, and yogurt will replenish a low zinc level. With cooking, there is a high loss of zinc. There are no specific storage sites in the body for zinc—which the body requires for about 200 reactions—therefore, supplementing with zinc is essential.

By the end of the eighteenth century, the British navy carried a mandatory supply of limes aboard ships to prevent the accursed disabling scurvy, symptoms of which were bleeding into the skin and mucous membranes, loose teeth, and spongy gums. This also is why the British are nicknamed limeys. Shortly thereafter, the Japanese provided their sailors with barley to ward off beri-beri, a disease of degenerative changes in the nerves, the digestive system, and the heart due to a lack of thiamine, a B vitamin.

The Polish biochemist, Casimir Funk, came up with the idea that foods contained vitamins (the name he invented for them). He believed that some diseases were caused by specific deficiencies, and that particular diseases could be prevented and overall health maintained by adding vitamin-rich foods to a diet. He named vitamins alphabetically, beginning with vitamin "B" for beri-beri. The later discovery of a vitamin necessary for coagulation led to vitamin K, with the "K" standing for *koagulation* (the German spelling).

A group of vitamins with similar properties and functions are called coenzymes. (An enzyme is a protein that promotes a chemical change in other substances or reactions, and remains unchanged in that process; a coenzyme is necessary for the enzyme to carry out its biochemical mission.) These coenzymes are the water-soluble B group of vitamins, which include biotin, choline, inositol, folic acid, niacin (vitamin B_3, which is now available in a more active form, a coenzyme known as NADH), pantothenic acid, para-aminobenzoic acid (PABA), pyridoxine hydrochloride (vitamin B_6), riboflavin (vitamin B_2), thiamine (vitamin B_1), as well as vitamins B_{12} (cyanocobalamin), B_{15} (pangamic acid), and B_{17} (amygdalin). All natural vitamins are considered organic because the basis for them is the element carbon. Humans cannot manufacture vitamin C (ascorbic acid), and your dog and cat do not require it (animals do not all need the same vitamins).

The way vitamins are stored depends on whether they are fat soluble or water soluble, meaning they will dissolve in either fat or water. The water-soluble vitamins, if in excess, are excreted in the urine. Excess fat-soluble vitamins, however, are stored in body fat.

Fat-Soluble Vitamins

I use my own mnemonic—ADEK—to remember which vitamins are fat soluble.

Vitamin A

Often used topically for the skin as a moisturizer in over-the-counter and prescription medications, vitamin A also aids in vision by feeding the rods in the back of the eye and making it possible to see in dim light. It also is effective in the growth of bones and teeth, and in keeping the reproductive and immune systems alert. Carotenoids—precursors to vitamin A—are found in the pigments of fruits and vegetables and then converted to vitamin A. Beta-carotene is a major source of vitamin A. New studies suggest that the carotenoids are effective in preventing or slowing macular degeneration.

As early as the fetal stage, vitamin A plays a crucial role in the development of the brain. In underdeveloped countries, the deficiency of this vitamin is a grave concern, affecting millions of children.

Food Sources: Apricots, carrots, mangos, papayas, pumpkins, spinach, and sweet potatoes.

Dosage: 5,000–10,000 IU a day; beta-carotene: 15 mg a day.

Vitamin D

This vitamin is required for the absorption of calcium, which is essential for strong bones and teeth. Calciferol, a form of vitamin D, occurs in fish oils and egg yolks. This is the form of the vitamin that is added to milk and margarine. Another form of this vitamin, cholecalciferol, is created when the ultraviolet rays of the sun react with chemicals under your skin. Vitamin D provides the proper balance for calcium and phosphorus to support the mineralization in bone.

Dosage: 400 IU a day.

Vitamin E

All beings, human and animal, require vitamin E for health. Its many benefits for heart disease include its acting as a mild anticoagulant. It protects the nerve membranes from free radicals, and when taken with vitamin A, it prevents damage from air pollution or other environmental toxins.

Vitamin E guards against cognitive decline and Alzheimer's disease. Many important studies, including the 1996 Cambridge University Study in England, have shown vitamin E to be vital in treating heart disease. People who have had a heart attack and then take 800 IUs of vitamin E are protected against a second heart attack. Another study from the University of Minnesota has shown that women sixty-five and older who take vitamin E supplements or get it from their diet reduce their risk of heart disease by 66 percent.

In 1997, *The New England Journal of Medicine* reported that vitamin E outperformed one of the leading drugs given to people for Alzheimer's disease. Also, diets rich in vitamin E reduce the risk of Parkinson's disease by an astonishing 61 percent. In those who already had Parkinson's disease, taking vitamin E along with vitamin C dramatically slowed the progress of this insidious disease.

Most vitamin E supplements consist of alpha-tocopherol, while foods are richer in gamma-tocopherol. These different forms of vitamin E oppose different types of free radicals.

Caution: High doses of vitamin E (2,000 IU per day) are associated with increased bleeding. Anyone on anticoagulants should check before supplementing with vitamin E, even in a much lower dose.

Food sources: Green leafy vegetables, nuts, vegetable oil, and whole grains.

Dosage: 400–800 IU per day, mixed tocopherols (natural).

Vitamin K

Vitamin K is essential for healthy bones because it activates necessary proteins that aid in the formation of new bone. And this fat-soluble vitamin helps produce specialized proteins in blood plasma, such as prothrombin (responsible for blood clotting). Although food sources are plentiful, most vitamin K is made from colonies of bacteria in the intestine.

Food sources: Broccoli, cabbage, cheese, dark leafy green vegetables, fruit, kale, lettuces, liver, spinach, and turnips.

Dosage: 65 mcg a day for females; 80 mcg a day for males.

Water-Soluble Vitamins

These vitamins dissolve in water; the body does not store them so they require constant replenishing. Any excess intake of water-soluble vitamins is excreted in urine.

B Vitamins

The B vitamins are also enormously important in preserving your health. Among their many functions, they help maintain optimal brain function by fighting homocysteine, a major risk factor for stroke and heart disease. Elevated homocysteine levels are irrevocably linked to brain disease, and specifically to:

- Cognitive decline

- Damaged blood vessels

- Loss of memory

- Neural degenerative disorders

Vitamin B₁ (Thiamine). This vitamin is required for the production of enzymes that convert glucose into energy for optimal brain function. It is involved in four different body processes that extract energy from carbohydrates. Thiamine is found in every body tissue, but its level is highest in the heart, kidneys, and liver.
    Food sources: Beans, fish, lean pork, liver, nuts, spinach, and unrefined cereals and grains.
    Dosage: 50 mg a day.

Vitamin B₂ (Riboflavin). This vitamin is necessary for the digestion of proteins and carbohydrates. It protects the health of the mucous membranes (moist tissues) of the body, helps produce more cellular energy, and enhances eye function.
    Food sources: Almonds, Brazil nuts, brewer's yeast, chicken, eggs, fish, and wheat germ.
    Dosage: 30 mg a day.

Vitamin B₃ (Niacin). This vitamin is important in producing cellular energy in the brain and throughout the body. Niacinamide, nicotinic acid, and nicotinamide are the same as niacin. Research has shown that niacin:

- Aids in fighting depression and short-term memory loss.

- Facilitates impulse transmission for proper brain functioning.

- Helps to assuage fatigue.

- Helps to regulate the metabolism and neuron oxygen supply.

- Improves the ratio of LDL (bad) and HDL (good) cholesterol (HDL and LDL are two different types of cholesterol—the ratio of the two predicts cardiac health).

- Lowers cholesterol.

    In a study done by Eli Lilly and the Oregon Health Sciences University, niacin caused an increase in homocysteine. This trial involved fifty-two patients who took niacin and a cholesterol-lowering drug, colestipol. The homocysteine levels in the plasma increased substantially (elevated levels are a risk factor for heart attacks and strokes). This small study was reported in *The American Heart Journal* in 1999 and has yet to be duplicated for validation. Niacin is, however, cardioprotective since it lowers LDL (bad) cholesterol and elevates HDL (good) cholesterol. If you take it, continue to take B_6, B_{12}, and folic acid, which will reduce homocysteine elevation.

Food sources: Beets, chicken, fish, peanuts, salmon, and tuna.

Dosage: 100 mg a day.

Vitamin B₅ (Pantothenic Acid). This vitamin is involved in more than one-hundred different metabolic processes, including energy metabolism, carbohydrates, lipids (fats), and proteins. It is also important in synthesizing neurotransmitters, including hemoglobin, lipids, serotonin, and steroid hormones. Low levels have been associated with burning feet syndrome—burning, aching feet and even excessive sweating (this occurs more in women). This syndrome may be experienced in diabetes, hypothyroidism, renal failure (dialysis patients), rheumatoid arthritis, and a vitamin-B deficiency.

Food sources: Avocado, lobster, poultry, soy, sweet potato, and yogurt.

Dosage: 75 mcg a day.

Vitamin B₆ (Pyridoxine). This vitamin is necessary for the synthesis and break-down of amino acids, the building blocks of protein. It aids in the formation of antibodies and red blood cells, as well as in the metabolism of fats and carbohydrates. Pyridoxine also reduces leg cramps and muscles spasms, and is involved in the balance of phosphorus in the body.

Food sources: Bananas, brewer's yeast, eggs, cabbage, meats, pecans, and wheat germ.

Dosage: 2 mcg a day.

Vitamin B₉ (Folic Acid, Folate). Folic acid is the synthetic form found in supplements. Folate occurs naturally. This water-soluble B vitamin is essential to brain health, but is not well stored in the body. Low concentrations of folic acid are associated with an increased risk of Alzheimer's disease and dementia. Researchers at the University of Kentucky reported that low folate levels are directly linked with a high degree of atrophy in the cerebral cortex. Folate is needed to make DNA and RNA, the building blocks of the cells, and have been shown to prevent changes in the DNA that could lead to cancer.

The intake of folate is crucial during periods of rapid cell division and growth, as in infancy and pregnancy, and an adequate intake of it is needed to prevent spina bifida, a neural-tube birth defect that results in a deformed spine. Broccoli, spinach, and other folate-rich foods do not, unfortunately, provide enough folate for the body, and folic acid in supplement form is, in fact, better absorbed than the natural food form.

A folate deficiency occurs with:

- Alcohol abuse

- Anemia

- Liver disease

- Medications, such as the anti-convulsants Dilantin or metformin for type 2 diabetes

- Methotrexate

- Pregnancy

- Renal dialysis

Note: Along with vitamins B_6 and B_{12}, folic acid is a member of a protective triad that will reduce homocysteine. All three B vitamins are crucial in the prevention of heart attacks and strokes.

Food sources: Avocado, beef liver, broccoli (boiled), chicken liver, lima beans, papaya, pinto beans, and spinach (boiled or raw). (A daily supplement is better absorbed than folate from food.)

Dosage: 400–800 mcg a day.

Vitamin B_{12} (Cobalamin or Cyanocobalamin). Of all the B vitamins, B_{12} is the most important for brain functioning, memory retention, and the production of myelin (nerve sheath), which protects the covering of neurofibers. The latest research indicates that individuals who have *H. pylori* stomach disease (a bacterial infection in the stomach associated with chronic ulcers and atrophy as well as chronic gastritis) can have a deficiency of B_{12}. When this stomach disease is eradicated, it eliminates the B_{12} deficiency. Vitamin B_{12} is required for normal nerve-cell activity and DNA replication. Many studies show that older people have a B_{12} deficiency, and may develop neuropsychiatric problems, including disorientation and confusion, which are often secondary effects of their inability to absorb B_{12} due to gastric atrophy. A deficiency of B_{12} can also lead to elevated homocysteine levels.

The question always is: Do vegetarians get enough B_{12}, since it is not found in plants? An Australian study reported in the *American Journal of Clinical Nutrition,* September 1999, found that as many as 73 percent of Australian vegetarians are deficient in B_{12}. It was recommended that their intake of this vitamin be increased by supplements of B_{12}, or foods fortified with it.

Frank Lederle, M.D., of the Minneapolis Veteran's Affairs Medical Center, emphasizes that physicians are not educated to the fact that *oral* B_{12} (cobalamin) works. As long as thirty years ago, research established that oral doses of 1 mg a day were effective in treating cobalamin-deficiency disorders. A deficiency of B_{12} often occurs without anemia, but since many doctors equate anemia with a deficiency of this vitamin, they do not know that the absence of anemia does not rule out this deficit.

Food sources: Animal food, including beef and liver, cheese, fortified cereals, and soy products.

Dosage: Injection: 1,000 mcg twice weekly for the first month, then twice monthly; Orally: Sublingual tabs 1,000 mcg a day.

Vitamin C

It would take many pages to list the numerous benefits of this widely used vitamin. It is involved in the maintenance and production of connective tissue, the largest amount of protein in the body. Wound healing requires vitamin C; it is a strong antioxidant protecting the immune system, and it is involved in some hormone synthesis.

Vitamin C was first isolated by a Hungarian biochemist and Nobel Prize winner, Dr. Szent-Györgyi, but Dr. Linus Pauling was the first to recognize its crucial role in helping to maintain and stimulate a healthy immune system by protecting against free radicals. Dr. Pauling recommended that vitamin-C intake should be 1,000 mg a day or more because that was the dosage required to completely saturate the blood plasma. If possible, take vitamin C in divided doses throughout the day.

The National Institute on Aging reported that older people who take vitamin C supplements have a 50 percent reduced risk of dying prematurely from disease than people who do not supplement with this vitamin. An Italian study concluded that older people, especially those who are sick, are exposed to a much higher level of oxidative stress than younger people. This is reflected in their low blood levels of vitamin C. Additional studies have shown that people with asthma, arthritis, cancer, diabetes, and heart disease have much lower levels of vitamin C than healthy people. What does that tell you? Could the keys to chronic degenerative disease, or even growing older, be a vitamin and mineral deficiency of massive proportions? Have you ever had a blood test that would show the level of the major vitamins and minerals in your blood?

Mathias Rath, M.D., who worked with Dr. Pauling and is a very pro-vitamin physician, has stated that such antioxidants as vitamins C, E, and beta-carotene may prove as potent as antibiotics and vaccines in fighting disease. Many studies show that people who maintain a good vitamin level can delay the onset and the severity, as well as the ravages, of chronic aging diseases. If you insist on eating bacon and sausage, you need to know that vitamin C can mimimize some of the damage from these foods because it helps prevent the sodium nitrite, a preservative in these meats, from reacting at high temperatures to form nitrosamines, which are deadly carcinogens.

Food Sources: Avocado, basil, beef, broccoli, Brussels sprouts, cauliflower, fish, fruits, kale, liver, mustard greens, onions (raw), papaya, parsley, peppers, poultry, squash, and vegetables.

Dosage: Minimum: 500 mg a day; Maximum: 2,000 mg (2 grams) a day or to bowel tolerance.

Vitamin H (Biotin)

Vitamin H is used in cell growth, and in the production and metabolism of fatty acids. The Krebs cycle is the biochemical pathway through which energy is released from food, and vitamin H is in that equation. A shortage of this vitamin has been associated with thinning hair. Researchers have found that biotin is helpful in maintaining a steady blood-sugar level. Bodybuilders or athletes who consume raw eggs may be deficient, as eggs prevent the absorption of biotin.

Food sources: Beef, cauliflower, cheese, chicken, liver, nuts, salmon, sardines, and spinach.

Dosage: 0.3 mg a day.

Vitamin P (Bioflavonoids)

This is not really a vitamin, but is usually listed as such because it is synergistic with Vitamin C. Vitamins P and C protect each other against oxidation, and, as with vitamin C, the body cannot manufacture bioflavonoids. Research has shown that biofavonoids are important in preserving capillary integrity by working with vitamin C to protect the thin-walled, smaller blood vessels and capillaries from bleeding and bruising. A diet that includes fruits and vegetables should provide sufficient amounts of bioflavonoids.

Food sources: Garlic, grapes, green tea, onions, oranges (white pulpy part), and red berries.

Dosage: 500 mg a day.

INTRODUCTION TO MINERALS

Minerals are inorganic substances of neither plant nor animal origin that are mined from the earth. Minerals are found in beans, dairy products, fruits, meat, nuts, and vegetables. At the very least, I recommend adding the minerals listed below to your vitamin supplements.

Magnesium

Every cell in our body requires this mineral. Half the magnesium in our bodies is in the cells. The other half is combined with calcium and phosphorus in the bones, with 1 percent found in the blood.

Low levels of magnesium are prevalent in people who take diuretics or have an intestinal malabsorption syndrome. Studies have shown that when animals are deficient in magnesium, they age rapidly and die earlier. People who are magnesium deficient tend to experience signs of old age earlier, including brain attacks, heart attacks, hypertension, insulin resistance, and obstructed blood vessels. The death of the mitochondria (the powerhouse of the cell) can result from inadequate levels because the heart is left unprotected against any developing coronary arterial spasm or abnormal heart rhythms, and this can lead to sudden death.

Magnesium inhibits the release of thromboxane, which makes blood platelets stickier and more prone to clotting. Keeping bones strong requires magnesium as well as calcium and vitamin D, so women with osteoporosis need to have their magnesium levels checked. The ratio of magnesium to calcium is important, since too much calcium can lead to heart attacks, more clot formation, and strokes. If you take the standard dose of 1,200 mg of calcium, you need 600 mg of magnesium.

Food sources: Cashews, hazelnuts, peanuts, pecans, pumpkins, pumpkin seeds, salmon, squash, tofu, and walnuts.

Dosage: 300–600 mg a day—the magnesium chloride or magnesium gluconate forms are absorbed well.

Selenium

This trace-mineral antioxidant is very powerful in supporting the immune system. It is necessary for the creation of glutathione peroxidase, an enzyme that quenches the free radicals that attack fat molecules. As people age, selenium levels fall, which leads to the risk of arthritis, cancer, and heart disease. Selenium is being studied intensively in cancer prevention because it is known to prevent mutations, as well help to repair damaged cells, thereby giving the immune system a boost.

A Finnish study reported that selenium reduces heart disease. It found that people with the lowest blood levels of selenium were three times more likely to die of heart disease than those with higher levels of selenium, and it also found that selenium prevented platelet aggregation. Low selenium levels may be a cause of hypothyroidism because this mineral is part of an enzyme responsible for the conversion of T4 (thyroxine) to T3 (triiodothyronine); T3 then converts to the active thyroid hormone in the bloodstream. Selenium may also help reduce arthritis symptoms.

Food sources: Beef, Brazil nuts, calves liver, plant foods, raw egg, seafood, and walnuts.

Dosage: Adults under sixty: 100 mcg a day; Over age sixty: 200 mcg a day.

Zinc

This important mineral plays a major role in protein formation and is needed for growth and maintenance of all tissues. Zinc is a component of many enzyme systems and is therefore involved in most metabolic processes. Zinc is often lost in cooking. Some cereals are fortified with zinc (read the labels).

Zinc helps stabilize cell membranes and is important in the immune-system pathways. Research has shown that one-third of supposedly healthy Americans over the age of fifty are deficient in zinc, and 90 percent of the older population does not supplement with zinc. Zinc can help keep the thymus gland active and therefore facilitate its connection with the immune system. Dr. A. Prasad at Wayne State University School of Medicine in Michigan believes that more than 20 million Americans are probably unknowingly at risk for infection and degenerative disease because of insufficient zinc in their diets. He found that by giving test subjects 30 mg of zinc gluconate daily for six months, their immune systems improved, as measured by the output of thymuline, a hormone critical to the formation of lymphocytes. And, in response to zinc, the production of interleukin-1 from the thymus doubled the production of T-cells, often forgotten antioxidants. Their deficiency has been associated with memory loss and disorientation.

Food sources: Cereals, lean meats, nuts, and seafood.
Dosage: 15–30 mg a day.

This vitamin and mineral section should help you make informed choices in your supplement plan and help you improve and sustain your health. The antioxidants in these supplements protect your brain and the DNA for every cell in your body, further strengthening your defense against the aging syndrome.

I believe aging is a disease that occurs because of depletion. For nonstop protection, the immune system requires constant boosting. Free radicals and oxidation cause changes in cells, which damage the DNA, and break down protein and cell membranes, creating a higher incidence of cancer, heart attacks, and strokes.

The recommended daily allowance (RDA) is now expanded by the dietary reference intakes (DRIs), which comprise four nutrient-based reference values, including RDA, adequate intake (AI), tolerable upper intake level (UL), and the estimated average requirement (EAR).

I find these values do not keep up with today's harried pace. People are primarily busier and cannot follow food value charts, so supplements should become a way of life, not as substitutes for foods, but as adjuncts to the diet to make up for any deficiencies. With the soil as nutrient depleted as it is, not to mention the further depletion of nutrients during the distribution of foods, it is unrealistic to consider eating eight bowls of spinach to obtain adequate nutrients from the vegetable, and supplements are clearly the answer here.

SPECIAL MIND BOOSTERS—SUPER ENERGIZERS FOR THE MIND

In addition to the vitamins and minerals I have put together for your brain health, there are special memory boosters I recommend to many of the patients I see in my office. You may think of these as supplementing your supplements. I call them *special mind boosters,* but they are actually super-energizers for the brain cells, and they enable people to formulate their thoughts faster over a longer period of time. While I don't believe that aging is always associated with a diminished thinking process—I know eighty-year-olds who possess a greater intellect and mental acuity than many lackluster college students—it is true that, as people age, energy production in the brain declines, and this can lead to a mental fatigue commonly known as brain fog. Plus, there is an attenuation of concentration, learning, and memory, and this age-related decline or mental cognitive impairment occurs as a result of diminishing neurons. By taking these mind-energizers or super antioxidants you can restore optimum function and vitality to your brain.

As people grow older, to forty-five or fifty years, the brain's energy production requires every possible boost from super nutrients. Energy is crucial to every cell in the body, but neurons require even more attention. Older is not always better, and a diminishing cellular function will contribute to age-related decline and brain fog. The major nutrients I have chosen here are important for energy production and mental clarity. The following four antioxidants give new meaning to the term brain food.

Acetyl-L-Carnitine

Carnitine is found in the brain, heart, muscles, and neural tissues, and in animal and dairy products. The structure of carnitine does not allow it to cross the blood-brain barrier, so acetyl-L-carnitine (ALC), which does cross the blood-brain barrier, becomes the activated form. Production of ALC decreases with age and it should be supplemented from age forty on to reverse cerebral aging. It is involved in energy production in the mitochondria and is needed for neurotransmitter synthesis. Neurons in the brain communicate with one another by releasing chemical messengers called neurotransmitters. There are more than one hundred neurotransmitters. Abnormalities in function can occur when substances, such as acetyl-L-carnitine, are deficient. Many neurological and psychiatric syndromes can result from deficient neurotransmission. Fat molecules are mobilized from the cell cytoplasm (substances outside the nucleus and mitochondria) and go through the mitochondrial membrane into the power plant for energy. ALC also removes waste from the mitochondria and helps make acetylcholine, a major neurotransmitter. It is involved in maintaining the cell membrane's integrity. ALC assists coenzyme Q_{10} (CoQ_{10}) and glutathione in protecting nerve cells against oxidative stress, and it has been successfully used in AIDS-related cognition decline and depression.

There is solid evidence that the neurodegenerative changes associated with brain aging may cause a decline in the neurochemicals known as nerve growth factor (NGF). The NGF primarily serves and supports cells in the hippocampus (the part of the temporal lobe where information is transferred into memory). Some studies have shown that ALC slows the deterioration of

Alzheimer's disease. And rat studies have demonstrated that when NGF was added to the ventricles (cavities) in the brain, where cerebrospinal fluid is made and circulates, it reversed both structural and behavioral deficits in aged rats. Although ongoing human studies have yet to be completed, scientists suspect it would work the same way in humans.

Food sources: Animal and dairy products.

Dosage: Not yet established (I personally take 1,200 mg per day).

Alpha-Lipoic Acid (ALA)

This energy booster, also known as thioacetic acid, is the only antioxidant that is both water and fat soluble, meaning it is available to all areas of the body. ALA is the agent that transforms glucose into energy in the mitochondria of the cells. And importantly, this booster can help restore the liver's most powerful antioxidant, glutathione (the subject of more than 40,000 articles in the Medline database).

Alpha-lipoic acid recycles vitamins C and E, and the coenzyme CoQ_{10}. It also significantly improves the tingling and painful numbness of the feet in people with diabetic neuropathy.

Food sources: Beef, brewer's yeast, broccoli, and spinach.

Dosage: 300–600 mg a day.

CoQ_{10} (Ubiquinone)

This is Japan's best-selling prescription drug for cerebrovascular disease. In the United States, you can purchase CoQ_{10} at any health food store. It is a powerful antioxidant and is synergistic with vitamin E. It also helps to recycle vitamins E and C. CoQ_{10} does occur naturally in all fruits and vegetables, but you can't get the full requirement without supplementation. It is an enzyme found in all the cells of the body, and is an important cofactor in the electron transport chain between cells. It is a vital component in the mitochondria (the cell's powerhouse), and if there is a decreased amount of CoQ_{10} in the cells, one of the body's most important sources of cellular energy is depleted.

Research sponsored by the National Institute of Neurological Disorders and Stroke found that 1,200 mg daily of CoQ_{10} slowed the progression of Parkinson's disease by 44 percent. According to Dr. M. Flint Beal, professor and chairman of the department of neurology at Cornell University Medical College in New York, "Research on CoQ_{10} must continue so that we may verify and move forward our current understanding of this powerful nutrient and its role within the human brain." It does not cross the blood-brain barrier readily, and aging, nutritional deficiencies, and statin drugs all decrease the body's natural CoQ_{10} production.

People who take statin drugs, such as Lipitor, Mevacor, or Pravachol, may experience a lack of energy secondary to the loss of CoQ_{10}, since these cholesterol-reducing drugs wash the CoQ_{10} out of the cells to the point of depletion. And sadly, too many doctors don't advise their patients that CoQ_{10} is crucial to proper heart functioning and should be supplemented.

CoQ_{10} improves cellular respiration, fights oxidative stress, and inhibits programmed cellular death (apoptosis). The brain is often susceptible to oxidative stress due to its high-fat content and rich oxygen supply. The accumulation of oxidative stress in the brain continues, with cell destruction, because it is normally low in antioxidant defense, so supplementation is important.

Does survival of the fittest mean survival for those who have the most antioxidants? For our brain survival and function, the answer is an unqualified *yes*.

As I said, brain vulnerability increases with age. In 1988, the National Institutes of Health (NIH) scientists recognized that excitotoxicity, which occurs in the brain, develops when the energy level of neurons decline. Stud-

CoQ10 Successes

Amy, a forty-eight-year-old graphic artist, had a mild case of chronic fatigue and a lack of focus in the morning through early afternoon. I put her on CoQ_{10} (60 mg), and was pleased when she told me that it gave her back her energy and she had a renewed ability to focus on her important projects. I hear this often from my patients.

George is seventy-two years old and had been taking several cardiovascular medications for years, including statin drugs, to reduce his high cholesterol. However, he complained regularly of fatigue and memory loss. After visiting many doctors, who recommended a multivitamin (containing either no CoQ_{10} or an insignificant 10 mg in the formula), George came to me and, upon my advice, now takes 100–200 mg of CoQ_{10} a day. This has helped him get back his energy and clarity of thought, and needless to say, he is delighted with this simple, effective solution to his problem.

ies show that CoQ_{10} protects against excitotoxicity by raising the cellular energy level. Newly published research suggests that CoQ_{10} can protect brain cells from chemicals, infections, neurotoxicity, and pesticides. CoQ_{10} fights aging and protects against the relentless oxidation of blood cholesterol, particularly LDL (bad) cholesterol.

Carl Folkers, Ph.D., director of the Institute for Biomedical Research at the University of Texas in Austin, has pioneered CoQ_{10} research since 1957. He found 25 percent less CoQ_{10} in the blood of people with heart disease than in the blood of healthy people. He also discovered 75 percent less CoQ_{10} in the heart tissue of people with heart disease, and found that 75 percent of the older population with cardiomyopathy (heart-muscle disease) improved after taking CoQ_{10}. Dr. Denham Harman of the University of Nebraska, the founder of the free-radical theory, said that CoQ_{10} is one of the few known antioxidants to penetrate and restore the vitality of the mitochondria.

Food sources: Beef, liver, and unprocessed grains. (Note: you cannot eat enough food stuff to obtain 100 mg a day.)

Dosage: 100 mg a day.

Nicotinamide Adenine Dinucleotide (NADH)

This is a coenzyme of the vitamin-B family (a coenzyme is the active or working form of a vitamin essential to metabolism). NADH converts the amino acid tyrosine into dopamine, which is important in Parkinson's disease and is involved in memory, concentration, and energy production.

NADH, a natural vitamin coenzyme found in the cells, is involved in multiple energy cycles involved in oxidizing (burning) food, including amino acids, carbohydrates, and fats, in order to produce adenosine triphosphate (ATP). This ATP energy is used by all cells in the body. Jorg Birkmayer, M.D. Ph. D., the first to discover the therapeutic application of NADH in cellular development and energy transmission, states, "NADH is the biological rocket fuel. It is the biological form of hydrogen, which reacts with oxygen present in our cells to produce energy. The more NADH we have, the more energy we can produce." The fundamental importance of NADH is its ability to convert food into energy. There have been no severe side effects reported with this supplementation.

The importance of ATP in muscle contraction and other cellular movements has been known for some time—the 1997 Nobel Prize in chemistry was based on the science related to the mechanism by which ATP shuttles energy.

Energy and the Coenzyme NADH

Laura, a sixty-year-old accountant and computer-science graduate of Stanford University, was diagnosed with chronic fatigue syndrome, a diagnosis which I doubted. She was dejected and had mild hypothyroidism, and I determined that by increasing her thyroid supplement she would improve. Six weeks later, after only a small improvement, I suggested to Laura that she also try 5 mg of NADH (ENADA) in the morning on an empty stomach. After one week on this supplement, the soreness in her muscles vanished and she told me she had more energy and focus than before. Two years down the road, Laura continues to do well, and is managing a sixteen- to eighteen-hour day. The best thing is that she has regained her confidence.

The key energy production influenced by NADH is in the brain and central nervous system. NADH stimulates cellular production of the neurotransmitters dopamine, noradrenaline, and serotonin, and the result is improved alertness, concentration, and mental clarity. It is also involved in the immune defense system. In AIDS-related mental decline, NADH has been helpful in enhancing memory and cognition. I take a 5 mg dose of NADH in the morning, and it has a positive effect on my energy level. I usually notice a boost in my vitality, clarity, and alertness within thirty minutes, and it lasts for most of the day; it's much more effective than drinking several cups of coffee.

Food sources: NADH occurs in cattle, fish, muscle, and poultry, but the absorption from these foods is miniscule; supplementation is recommended.

Dosage: Five (5) mg a day on an empty stomach; the dosage may be repeated two hours after lunch.

MIND BOOSTERS DERIVED FROM HERBS AND PLANTS

Plant-based supplements are a vital facet of optimum health care.

Ginkgo Biloba

Extracted from the leaves of the ginkgo biloba, the oldest tree in the world, this herb has been used in China for thousands of years. Even so, it took a long time for Chinese herbal practitioners to get around to discovering it, as the ginkgo tree has been on the planet for at least 200 million years. According to the classic Chinese pharmacopeia (a compendium of herbs), ginkgo has historically proved effective in treating cognitive decline. Ginkgo biloba is composed of flavonoids (also found in fruits and vegetables), which are powerful antioxidants with a positive influence on the immune system. Quercetin is arguably the most effective flavonoid in ginkgo. The active ingredients are enhanced when taken in combination with ascorbic acid—vitamin C (taking vitamin C daily covers you in this area).

In many people, ginkgo's beneficial effects begin in three to four weeks. Ginkgo biloba:

- Enhances the ability to focus.

- Increases the blood flow to the brain.

- May be helpful to people with Alzheimer's or Parkinson's disease.

- May help to avert a decline in eyesight.

- Prevents strokes and the clumping of red blood cells.

- Reduces oxidative damage to neurons.

- Serves as an anti-inflammatory agent.

- Slows cognitive decline.

Dosage: 120 mg a day.

Ginkgo Biloba and Tinnitus

Bill, a retired business executive, complained of tinnitus (ringing in the ears), which began slowly and became more frequent over the course of six months to the point where it was constant. This condition is usually attributed to atherosclerosis of the blood vessels supplying the inner ear. I placed him on a 60 mg dose of ginkgo and instructed him to take this two to three times a day. Within one week, he remarked that the annoying tinnitus had greatly diminished, and after one month, his symptoms had completely disappeared. As an additional benefit, Bill also noted an improved ability to focus.

Ginseng

Ginseng, in one or another of its forms, is perhaps the most widely used herb of all. The varieties sold in North America are American, Asian (Panax ginseng), and Siberian. Of these, the Asian version is, by far, the most stimulating and has been used in traditional Chinese medicine for millennia.

Ginseng is made up of saponins, emulsifying agents (a wetting agent) that have been used in Asia for centuries to treat circulatory diseases of the heart and brain. It has also been shown to inhibit fat oxidation in cardiac muscle and the liver. Ginseng decreases blood coagulation and levels of glucose, and research suggests that ginseng reduces cholesterol. Ginseng:

- Augments energy.

- Enhances the learning process.

- Improves memory.

- Provides mental clarity.

Dosage: 200 mg in the morning two to three times a week.

Huperzine A

Huperzine A is derived from the Chinese club moss plant. It is an acetylcholinesterase inhibitor. It inhibits the breakdown of the neurotransmitter acetylcholine, giving it a longer life span to allow muscles and organs to relax. Huperzine A has been shown to have major cognition-enhancing powers. A 1997 research paper by Robert Skolnick in *The Journal of the American Medical Association* *(JAMA)* discussed huperzine A as a possible herbal therapy for Alzheimer's disease. Additional studies on the subject are currently underway. Huperzine A:

- Enhances learning ability and memory.

- Heightens production of dopamine and norepinephrine neurotransmitters.

- Improves reaction time and cognitive processing in healthy individuals.

- Increases circulation to and in the brain.

Dosage: 200 mcg a day in divided doses (recommended particularly for people with moderately severe dementia).

Warning: Anyone who has been diagnosed with psychotic disorders should not take this drug.

Vinpocetine

This is an extract of the periwinkle plant. It is an herb that has proven effective for people with strokes. Vinpocetine:

- Blocks calcium from overpowering the damaged cells.

- Dilates blood vessels.

- Has blood-thinning potential.

- Is a cognitive enhancer.

- Speeds up the use of glucose and oxygen in the brain.

Dosage: 5 mg, two to three times a week.

NOOTROPICS—AKA SMART DRUGS

This umbrella term is used for a new class of drugs that act as cognitive enhancers. Nootropics (from *noose,* meaning mind, and *tropion,* translated as toward) have been called smart drugs because of the boost they provide to the brain. This is because they provide an increase of blood flow to the brain and also increase the levels of neurotransmitters, which actively contribute to memory and learning.

Dimethylaminoethanol (DMAE)

This chemical, produced naturally in the human brain, is used as a supplement to convert choline into the neurotransmitter acetylcholine. It has been beneficial in slowing age-related cognitive decline. DMAE:

- Diminishes the effects of attention-deficit disorder (ADD) in children and adults.

- Elevates mood.

- Enhances memory.

- Improves focus and alertness in young people.

- Promotes clarity of thought.

- Repairs damaged cell membranes.

- Reverses aging spots in the brain.

   Dosage: 100–300 mg a day.

Hydergine

This is a brand name for a combination of ergot-derivative drugs that are extracted from the ergot fungus of rye plants and prescribed to enhance cognition. Hydergine was discovered by a chemist, Dr. Albert Hoffman, who is more famous for the development of another ergot derivative—LSD. Hydergine:

- Enhances learning ability and memory.

- Heightens production of dopamine and norepinephrine—neurotransmitters that are powerful antioxidants.

- Improves reaction time and cognitive processing in healthy individuals.

- Increases blood flow to and in the brain.

   Dosage: 3–6 mg a day.
   Note: This drug requires a prescription. Studies in Europe used 9–12 mg a day. Hydergine is approved by the FDA for use in senile dementia.
   Warning: People who have been diagnosed with psychotic disorders should not take this drug.

Piracetam

Since 1970, the drug piracetam has been used in Europe as a prescription for dementia. While there is no conclusive proof of its effectiveness for humans, in laboratory studies, piracetam's power on aging rats has been exceptionally strong. Human studies are still being carried out, but it is believed that piracetam is most effective on people who have low levels of acetylcholine in their brains, and it may have some soothing ability in those who have recently had a stroke (further studies have shown a 19 percent improvement in those who have taken this drug). According to Belgian neurologist, Dr. Peter Paul

DeDeynd, piracetam may make the difference between being able to function independently at home or having to live in a nursing home. This is a powerful result that certainly warrants further study. Piracetam:

- Enhances microcirculation (blood flow in the brain).

- Fuels the creative process in some individuals.

- Increases production of adenosine triphosphate (ATP).

- Increases protein synthesis, thus aiding long-term memory.

- Is beneficial to cells that store and generate energy in the brain.

- May improve mental function.

This drug is not sold in the United States, but can be obtained in Mexico through foreign pharmacies.

Dosage: 400–800 mg tablets, up to 2,400 mg a day.

S-Adenosylmethionine (SAM-e)

This substance is not found in food. It is formed from methionine, an amino acid, and adenosine triphosphate (ATP). ATP is the body's cellular energy supply and is involved in at least forty vital biochemical processes. It is also essential to the formation of glutathione, a major antioxidant.

Depression can be a result of low levels of SAM-e. Deficient levels are often found in older depressed individuals and those with Alzheimer's disease. Dr. Richard Brown of Columbia University College of Physicians and Surgeons in New York, who is the coauthor of *Stop Depression Now,* has said that SAM-e is the best antidepressant he has ever prescribed.

SAM-e works faster than conventional antidepressants. By supplementing with SAM-e, you help increase the level of neurotransmitters in your brain, as well as the number of receptors that receive chemical messengers from them.

Dosage: 400 mg a day (enteric-coated is preferred).

SMART BRAIN FATS

The human brain is made up of 60 percent fat. Myelin, which is 75 percent fat, surrounds the axons, or fibers, of nerve cells and is involved in the speed of neural transmission. Fluctuations in fatty acids occur all through life and have a profound effect on the brain, particularly areas involving behavior, cognition, mood, and the sensation of having fluid movements (as in dancing).

Alpha-Glycerophosphocholine (GPC)

GPC is present in all cells of the body and tissues. Although the body produces GPC, the excessive demand for it in today's information age creates a need for more production or supplementation. GPC is a major source of choline, an essential nutrient important for renewal and repair. Choline is utilized in the production of acetylcholine, a major neurotransmitter. GPC is the active choline for the brain, since it raises the brain's choline level to support the production of ACH when a major demand for it occurs in the brain. Scientific studies have suggested an increased mental performance following supplementation with alpha-glycerophosphocholine—electroencephalographic (EEG) studies reveal improvement in electrical patterns in middle-aged and young healthy brains. GPC has been used in studies on stroke recovery and postheart surgery, as well as vascular dementia, and has demonstrated an ability to improve cognition and mood. Ongoing studies show an increase in growth hormone levels after GPC supplementation, as well as its beneficial effect on thyroid-stimulating hormone.

Dosage: 250 mg, twice a day.

Arachidonic Acid (AA)

One-third of brain fat is polyunsaturated. The most abundant of the fats are arachidonic acid and DHA. AA is an omega-6 fatty acid that is readily available in dairy products and meats. It must, however, be kept in balance with omega-3 fatty acids, or it will stimulate an excess production of inflammatory prostaglandins, which are derivatives of fatty acids. (A serious problem with the standard American diet, or SAD, and its overload of processed foods containing omega-6 fatty acids.) AA is a constituent of phospholipids in the cell membrane.

Dosage: AA is incorporated in phospholipids and is not taken by itself.

Docosahexaenoic Acid (DHA)

DHA is concentrated at the synaptic junction between the axons and dendrites (the synapse is where the communication between nerve cells—neurons—takes place). The other important location for DHA is in the mitochondria (powerhouse) within the neurons.

It is also present in the light receptors of the eyes. DHA is necessary for rhodopsin, a protein in the retinal rod cells that aids in the perception of light for visual function. DHA is found throughout the cerebral cortex and is crucial for brain development from fetus through childhood. It is important in pregnant women, nursing mothers, and vegetarians. Breastfeeding assures more critical fat absorption for a baby's body than cow's milk or formula—there is a relationship between adequate intake of DHA and our intelligence from infancy on. As reported by Michael A. Schmidt in his book *Smart Fats,* adults with a low level of DHA have a greater potential to develop dementia in their senior years. Low levels are also considered an important risk for Alzheimer's disease.

Dosage: 500 mg a day.

Phosphatidylcholine (PC)

While phosphatidylserine (PS) contains the amino acid serine, choline in PC is a precursor of acetylcholine, which is the brain's most important neurotransmitter. During pregnancy, choline is necessary in utero. When the fetus has an insufficient amount, poor brain development occurs. The B-complex vitamins that contain choline provide the brain with the ability to manufacture phosphatidylcholine and acetylcholine. Both are purified extracts from lecithin and are beneficial in depression, memory loss, and liver health. PC is responsible for maintaining the cell membrane. Phosphatidylcholine:

- May help assuage the effects of Alzheimer's disease.

- Provides normal brain development to the fetus.

Dosage: 120 mg, three times a day.

Phosphatidlyserine (PS)

This is the major phospholipid in the brain. Along with other phospholipids, it forms the basic structural component of cell membranes. It regulates the cell contents and has a role in providing the surface for receptors and enzymes. PS enhances cell-to-cell communication and the transfer of biochemical messages into brain cells. Phosphatidlyserine:

- Augments cognitive skills.

- Eases the learning process.

- Improves concentration.

- Protects cells from damage by free radicals.

Dosage: 300 mg a day.

REGIMEN FOR BRAIN-BOOSTER SUPPLEMENTS— SUPER ENERGIZERS FOR THE MIND

The following lists include the most important supplements to be taken daily, unless otherwise noted. Dosages are meant to be used as guidelines only and may vary according to your daily routine and individual needs. If, for example, you feel a cold coming on, you can boost the vitamins A and C, and the mineral zinc. In all cases, it may take a trial-and-error adjustment for individual brain chemistry.

Ages Twenty-Five to Forty

- Acetyl-L-carnitine: 300–600 mg

- Alpha-lipoic acid: 300–600 mg

- B-complex: 50 mg

- CoQ_{10}: 100–160 mg

- Fish oil capsule, includes omega-oils, EPA, DHA: 1,000 mg

- High-potency multivitamin/mineral, natural supplements to be taken five to seven times weekly

- NADH: 5 mg in the morning on an empty stomach

- Pantothenic acid: 250–500 mg

Ages Forty to Sixty

In this age span, hormone levels are beginning to decrease, along with energy and libido. A hormonal evaluation, in conjunction with supplements, is indicated. It is also recommended that the amount of carbohydrates be curbed at lunch in order to avoid the afternoon slump (carbohydrates make you sleepy).

- Acetyl-L-carnitine: 300–600 mg

- Alpha-lipoic acid: 600 mg (can be taken on different days but at least three times a week)

- B-complex: 50 mg

- CoQ$_{10}$: 160–200 mg

- DHEA: 25 mg for women (blood test required); 50 mg for men

- Fish oil: 1,000 mg

- Flaxseed oil: 1 teaspoon

- Ginkgo biloba: 60 mg twice a day, with breakfast and lunch

- Ginseng (Asian): 200 mg, two to three times a week

- High-potency multivitamin/mineral

- NADH: 5 mg in the morning on an empty stomach

- Testosterone: dosage depends on blood test

- Vitamin C: 1,000 mg

- Vitamin E: 400–800 IU

Ages Sixty Forward

Special attention is needed for this age group since many older people have medical conditions requiring additional prescription drugs, and some of them exacerbate the loss of thoughtful cognition. Depression, diabetes, thyroid disease, and a deficiency of B$_{12}$ will have negative brain effects. Anticoagulants for heart problems and drugs for hypertension also influence all supplementation.

- Acetyl-L-carnitine: 1,000 mg

- Alpha-lipoic acid: 300 mg twice a day

- B-complex: 50 mg

- CoQ$_{10}$: 200 mg

- Fish oil: 1,000 mg

- Ginkgo biloba: 120 mg, if not on blood thinners

- High-potency multivitamin/mineral

- NADH: 5 mg in the morning on an empty stomach

- Phospholipids: GPC: 250 mg twice a day; PC: 120 mg; PS: 300 mg

- Vitamin C: 1,000 mg

- Vitamin E: 400–800 IU, if not on blood thinners

Note: It is important to have your healthcare practitioner request a hormonal evaluation. Additional supplements should be considered with Alzheimer's or Parkinson's disease.

A Regimen Too Far

Eric, a thirty-three-year-old man who has trained as a bodybuilder for years, came to see me once or twice a year since experiencing a minor muscle injury. He had self-discipline, a strong desire to be a national champion, and a roomful of trophies, which he began acquiring when he won his first prize at age fourteen. The intensity of his focus kept his diet in balance, and he felt that adding supplements would give him an edge.

Some months ago, Eric came to me because he had the sudden onset of a severe headache, preceded by a weakness on his left side. Upon examination, I determined that as a result of his regimen, which had included high doses of aspirin, ginkgo biloba, occasional St. John's Wort, and vitamin E, all clotting inhibitors, he had developed a small hemorrhage in his brain. His dosage had been way out of range, and as soon as he stopped it, he made a good recovery. The point here is that aspirin and prescription medications may cause bleeding because they negatively affect clotting, and even supplements can be life-threatening when taken to the extreme. If you feel your dosage is out of balance, you may want to discuss it with your healthcare practitioner.

IN SUMMATION

This chapter is a guideline to some of the supplements that will make a difference in your degree of wellness and brain health. You might want to share this information with your nutritionally aware healthcare practitioner so that he or she can help you choose what is right for you. Alternating some of the vitamins, minerals, and smart drugs is one way to do it. I personally take thirty to thirty-six supplements a day because I believe they are essential to many chemical reactions in our cells and enzyme systems. The overused and outdated phrase *well-balanced diet* is not enough. I carry my supplements to the office during the week and always drink water throughout the day. No one should take all her or his supplements at the same time—for better absorption, they should be dispersed throughout the day.

CHAPTER 8

Environmental Toxins: The Enemies You Should Know

The brain—a pink pulsating membranous mass of twists and convulsions—innocence and genius together ensconced in a thick bony skull, surrounded, and protected, by a moat called the dura mater; hard mother. The primary organ of survival, it thrives on oxygen and glucose. In any polluted air of smoke, tar, burning fumes, or chemical/pesticide toxins it can never be at its peak function. If our body is the temple, then indeed the brain is its omniscient master and we must pay homage to it.

—GALE WISEMAN DAVIS

In 1954, Rachel Carson stated, "The more clearly we can focus our attention on the wonders and realities of the universe, the less taste we shall have for destruction." Her words ring true today. Our environment is toxic. The water we drink, the food we eat, the air we breathe is more contaminated now than at any time in the history of mankind. Amazingly, more of this damage has happened in the past ten decades than in the millions of years that preceded the beginning of the twentieth century.

Until the advent of the Industrial Revolution, the world was a wonderfully pure place with the air and water clear and the food supply untainted by pollution or chemicals of any kind. Ironically, it was due to man's desire to progress that much of his own environment was destroyed. Although life is easier today than a century ago, the chemically altered environment has caused irreversible disease to many who live on the planet.

Oncologists say 80 percent of all cancers are a direct response to chemical pollution of air, water, and food supplies. While the percentage may surprise you, I doubt the basic supposition will. Most of you know the effects on unborn fetuses from public health hazards, as evinced in Chernobyl in the Ukraine or the Love Canal tragedy in upstate New York.

Just as oncologists have warned of the relationship between environmental toxins and cancer, so many neurosurgeons have documented the inextricable relationship between a hazardous environment and brain disease. The incidence of primary brain tumors is now 12 per 100,000 people in the United States, and the number of people worldwide who die from brain tumors has increased 300 percent in some areas. Brain tumors are now the second leading cause of cancer deaths for children under nineteen years of age. And this year, approximately 17,200 people will be diagnosed with a brain tumor, which is twice as many as thirty years ago.

Toxins directly affecting the nervous system are known as neurotoxins, and they stem from the 1.9 billion pounds of chemicals dumped annually into America's air and water supplies. This information comes directly from the Environmental Protection Agency (EPA), a misnamed organization because, instead of providing protection, the EPA, over the course of a year, is allowing an additional 2.4 billion pounds of chemicals to be released into the atmosphere of planet Earth. There are approximately 70,000 synthetic chemicals in commercial use now, and most have not been tested for human safety.

Neurotoxins are very much the deleterious unknown enemies because many of them, such as cadmium, lead, mercury, and numerous pesticides, are colorless and odorless. The senses can't detect them.

Neurotoxicity is the direct effect of chemical exposure on the structure and function of the central and peripheral nervous system. The nerve cells are chemically damaged and the very sensitive myelin, a soft, white, fatty sheath around the core of a nerve fiber, becomes degraded, which impedes nerve conduction. The myelin sheath is actually a non-water-soluble tubular envelope, and its purpose is to speed the transmission rate of an electrical impulse along the axon. But the neurotoxins slow the transmission rate of the impulse, and the end result is a dysfunction of the nerves and brain, leading to poor mental development and behavioral problems.

Symptoms of neurotoxicity include:

- Impairment of the autonomic nervous system
- Loss of cognition
- Loss of motor control
- Tremors
- Weakness

Note: The autonomic nervous system regulates involuntary actions; most of its functions are on the subconscious level.

How toxic is our environment? Many people who lived through the 1960s believed a new day would come when consumer safety and human concerns would prevail, but regretfully this has not happened. Although small sparks of hope flicker occasionally, the apathy of the American public still seals our fate. Congress and the Senate continue to place business ahead of people, and with this myopia the environment may well have to reach a crisis point before our government takes an active forward position. That is why people need to wake up. Health, like hygiene, has to begin at home, and people can't continue to wait for someone else to take the initiative while the toxins take over and become more pervasive. It's like putting up a traffic light after the collision.

If this sounds rather grim, that's because it is, but there are serious steps you can take to secure your brain health against environmental toxins. The first thing is to follow the nutritional and supplement plans I discussed in Chapters 6 and 7. Your health will be renewed by removing the poisons from your system, and you will make a grand leap toward reversing the effects of toxic exposure every day.

Since it is virtually impossible to avoid being exposed indoors or outside to industrial pollutants, the best thing you can do is be keenly aware and reduce your exposure to them at school, work, and especially in your own home. By actively avoiding environmental health hazards and minimizing toxic accumulation you will be the guardian of your brain cells and prevent disease.

TOXINS IN THE HOME

Would you believe that the air in your own home can be more hazardous to your health than the air you breathe outdoors, and that your routine domestic activities can release pollutants that place your brain health at risk? Believe it because air-conditioning units, electrical heating, and the tasks of cleaning and cooking can all serve as media for the spread of bacteria and pollutants that challenge even the healthiest people. And these effects are even more pronounced in infants and young children whose immune systems are not fully developed, or in older people who may experience chronic illnesses or feel the general effects of aging and failing health.

These biological pollutants that wreak such havoc on health are living organisms that float through the air or live on surfaces within the home.

These home-based pollutants negatively affect your brainpower and health just as smoke-related lung disease can lead to poor brain performance because of the body's reduced capacity to replace carbon dioxide in the blood with new supplies of oxygen. This creates an imbalance, which will lead to biochemical changes in the brain, and decades of exposure to the pollutants can result in reduced mental functioning and diminished longevity.

Many of my patients bristle at the suggestion that their homes are unclean or unsafe in any way. I can understand this—as the saying goes, "cleanliness is next to godliness," and no one wants to be thought of as either a shoddy housekeeper or someone who doesn't do the best for his or her family. But even the most meticulous, fastidious people cannot combat certain household pollutants unless they are curious about them and want to know more about what they are.

Among the most pervasive and pernicious household foes are:

- Animal dander

- Bacteria and viruses

- Dust mites

- Mold or other fungi (dust on clothing)

- Pollen

The Downside of Home-Cleaning Chemicals

Michael, a forty-seven-year-old salesman, spent a quarter of a century selling cleaning supplies for the home. Every week he drove long distances to different states with many varieties of these industrial chemicals, and being in contact with them for long periods of time continually exposed him to them. These toxic supplies eventually took their toll and he developed a chronic cough, fever, and ongoing fatigue. After several visits to his primary care physician, and a complete blood workup, Michael was diagnosed with myelogenous leukemia, a fatal blood disorder attributed to the noxious chemicals he had been exposed to over the years. This cautionary tale has an unfortunate conclusion that can be avoided by paying closer attention to the chemicals around you in your life.

Some of you with allergies, asthma, or allergic reactions to any of the above culprits may already know about these biological pollutants in your home, which may already be doing damage to you in the form of lost school or work days, or general malaise. I believe that much of what is commonly diagnosed as chronic fatigue syndrome can be traced to environmental allergens that have not been properly identified by either the person or her or his physician.

How Are Environmental Toxins Spread in the Home?

Studies show that up to 50 percent of all existing household structures have damp conditions that encourage the growth of biological pollutants that, in most cases, are living organisms. So how can you tell if you are having any reactions to these household pollutants? Since most reactions are allergic in nature, you may have experienced one or more of the following symptoms:

- Coughing
- Fatigue
- Headache
- Incessant sneezing
- Itching, red, or watery eyes
- Nasal congestion
- Shortness of breath
- Wheezing

Many people believe they just have to live with these symptoms. This is never a good thing. First of all, no one should have to go through life with any condition that is harmful, rather than treat or avoid it. Second, these symptoms may actually be indications of toxic reactions that can cause long-term damage to many or all organs of the body, notably the brain and the liver.

The good news is that no one is helpless in the fight against these unseen destroyers. Whether you feel perfectly healthy or are aware that you have negative reactions to environmental pollutants, I strongly recommend that you take steps to make sure your home is as safe from these pollutants as possible. This will take some time, but isn't your brain worth it? I believe the effort you put into this project will save the wear and tear on your immune system and have positive consequences for your family's long-term health.

Here are the most prevalent environmental toxins in your home and how to control them.

Carpets

New chemicals in carpets are major sources of noxious emissions containing volatile organic compounds. But that's just the beginning—the installation material itself (padding, adhesives, etc.) causes allergic reactions, notably fatigue, in a number of my patients. If you think your carpet is a clean part of your residence, it isn't. You are providing a home for a whole host of biological pollutants that include dust mites, fungi, and pesticides. Since arming yourself with knowledge is your best defense, I suggest the following course of action.

• Be aware. When purchasing a new carpet, select one with the lowest possible emission standards (your dealer and the EPA website will have information on this subject).

• Leave your home during the carpet installation. Allow the maximum time for fresh air to enter your house, turn on your ceiling fan, open doors and windows during installation, and do not return until the air has had a chance to clear after the installation.

• Set your air-conditioning unit to the exhaust function and leave it on as long as possible so that toxins from the carpet are circulated to the outside of your dwelling.

• Maintain your carpet using the safest possible products and processes (instead of carpet cleaners or powders, use water and Ivory soap, for example).

Recently, the British Broadcasting Company (BBC) produced a program about carpet toxicity, in which John Roberts, an American environmental engineer, was interviewed by *The New Scientist* magazine. He discussed the high level of heavy metals, hydrocarbons, pesticides, and polychlorinated biphenols (PCBs) in carpets. His conclusion was that carpets are the largest reservoir of dust in the house and therefore need frequent vacuuming.

Another expert, Robert Lewis of the EPA, stated that long-banned pesticides can reside in carpet dust because carpets are not subject to rain and sun, or other outside forces which can break down pollutants. The EPA found that the level of pesticides in homes was increased four hundred–fold by contamination brought in on the feet of people and the paws of pets.

Combustible Gases and Materials

These gases can be insidious agents. In this category, fireplaces are considered the most harmful indoor-air contaminants, since they produce carbon monoxide from incomplete combustion. This is true whether you are burning wood, natural gas, coal, or oil. To prevent this, one good solution is to use only a sealed combustion process (glass doors) in your fireplace that allows you to enjoy watching the fire without breathing it in.

Dust

Mites live in dust and are not visible to the human eye. Most homes have dust-mite infestation—there are billions of them living in our homes—and they thrive in bedding, drapes, fabrics, sofas, Venetian blinds, and wallpaper (as gory as it sounds, dust mites subsist on skin particles from humans).

Mites also live deep down in carpets and cannot be removed by everyday vacuuming. If you are seriously allergic to mites, you may have to use washable area rugs rather than wall-to-wall carpet.

Dust has serious ramifications for brain health. Along with mold, it accounts for 14 million physician visits per year to treat major health manifestations, such as asthma, cough, fatigue, fever, headache, lethargy, and poor concentration.

Metal Pollution

Until the extremely toxic lead-based paints were banned by the federal government in 1978, they were used to decorate many homes, inside and out, and their long-lasting effects are everywhere—in the soil around the homes, in household dust, and in the air that circulates throughout the homes. If you are living in an older home where lead pipes were used, it's especially important that you drink bottled or filtered water, as the water from the faucet has come through lead paint and lead pipes. In addition, lead contamination can come from chewing on pencils, hobbies (stained-glass making, furniture refinishing, pottery crafting, etc.), and painted toys and furniture.

An estimated 900,000 American children between the ages of one and five have dangerous levels of lead in their bodies. Even children who appear strong and healthy can have a toxic burden of lead, which has deleterious effects on the brain and nervous system. Lead's widely publicized damages to a child's body can be devastating and, depending on the severity of the lead poisoning, symptoms from exposure to lead can include:

- Dramatic hyperactivity

- Headaches

- Inability to focus

- Learning problems

- Poor memory

- Stunted growth

These problems are not limited to children, however. Lead is also extremely harmful to adults and can cause reproductive problems for both men and women. In the most serious cases, infertility is the result. The brain is also very vulnerable, since poor memory and concentration can also result from lead toxicity.

A study by the Harvard School of Public Health concurs. It showed that individuals with higher-than-average levels of lead in their bones had abnormally low levels of hemoglobin and red blood cells, which suggests that lead stored in bones can also exert a toxic effect, even when it's not present in the blood. Although additional studies need to be done, there is ample medical basis for the belief that lead in the bones or blood can cause cognitive deficiencies in teenagers and adults.

A prominent researcher, Howard Hu, associate professor of occupational medicine at Harvard, has stated, "If lead can affect an enzyme system involving the production of hemoglobin with this level and sensitivity, you must wonder whether it is affecting similar enzyme systems in the brain." It is. Every marker indicates that lead interferes with the chemical production that occurs in the brain.

Moisture

The problem of moisture inside the home can be rampant or nearly nonexistent, depending on the area of the country. As you would imagine, this is a major problem in humid areas, such as subtropical Florida, the coastal areas of the Gulf of Mexico, and Georgia. There is, of course, much less moisture in such desert regions as Arizona and New Mexico.

The first thing to do to eliminate the moisture is make sure there are no building materials strewn in or around your home. Firewood should not be left out uncovered to fester. If you smell a musty or dank odor, you can be sure some kind of toxin is lurking—damp areas are primary breeding grounds for the worst kinds of biological agents (in terms of flora and fauna, they're not dissimilar from a swamp or dumping ground). Moreover, if you live in a part of the country where houses are traditionally made of wood, as in northern California, your family's home may be an ecosystem for unseen flora and fauna.

If you can smell or see fungi in one or more areas of your home or apartment, it is obligatory that you treat this situation seriously—or move. There are many qualified professionals who deal with these problems. If you elect to rid your home of the toxins yourself, I recommend you visit the Environmental Protection Agency's website www.epa.gov/ which has much excellent information on this subject.

Mold

Mold contamination has become a legal and financial nightmare in the United States—at present there are more than 10,000 mold-related lawsuits pending. The debate about mold's effect on our health, specifically on brain health, rages on, with advocates on both sides of the issue vehemently defending their positions. As William Baker, M.D., an assistant professor and allergy specialist at the Indiana University School of Medicine says, "mold is everywhere, and is the most common life form in the world." Dr. Baker claims that there is no proven causative effect between mold and memory loss.

Other researchers, however, including Helene Uhlman, the administrator of the Hammond Indiana Health Department, has said, "Concerns about the health effects of toxic mold are not overblown." She has found, for example, that a small group of black molds emits chemicals called mycotoxins, which become airborne and can have seriously deleterious effects on human brain health.

Exactly how dangerous mold is depends on its size and manifestation. Typically, the danger level occurs when it reaches proportions of two square feet or larger. Also, if mold has infested dry wall, insulation, and/or carpeted areas, take measures to remove it. You can find mold experts on the web to consult with, and they can guide you accordingly.

Pet Sprays

"Safe for humans," the labels on animal-care products audaciously proclaim. I vigorously disagree. Insecticidal flea and tick shampoos, sprays, and dips have been shown to be toxic, not only to pests, but to your pets and you. A pesticide collar, for example, emits a toxic cloud inhaled by both your pet and everyone else in the household. Moreover, veterinarians who have been in practice for several decades report that compared to preceding years, in the past twenty years there has been a higher incidence of serious, often inexplicable, health problems in animals of all kinds.

In her mid-twentieth-century book, *Silent Spring*, Rachel Carson, the prescient and extraordinary environmentalist, wrote that pets and wildlife are subjected to a toxic environment even greater than that of humans because they are closer to nature than humans. In spite of ridicule by big business and an unbelieving public, Rachel Carson spent much of her career warning North Americans of the health threats brought on by widespread use of chemical pesticides. Her pioneering efforts helped to create the Environmental Protection Agency (EPA) in 1970, which subsequently banned the highly toxic pesticide DDT in 1972.

Volatile Organic Compounds

Just about every house in North America contains paints, stains, glues, petrochemical-based compounds, adhesives, and other materials that are rife with carcinogens. After these chemicals are opened and used in the home, they're released into the atmosphere, where they combine with ozone and are carried far and wide into the environment.

If you must keep these toxic pollutants in or near your living space, make sure they are kept in an area not frequented by children or others with unformed or compromised immune systems. Make sure these volatile compounds are all capped, sealed, and kept outside of the house at all times, not in an attic, basement, or utility area that are just other rooms in the house.

TOXINS AT WORK
Sick Building Syndrome

The term *sick building syndrome* (SBS) refers to a condition in which occupants of a building experience health effects from spending time in the building.

Toxins in Artist's Studio

Blair has been a successful painter since childhood. She began with finger painting, and over the years has become an internationally known artist. Her theme is color, color everywhere. Spray paint is often her medium and she rarely bothered to use a mask as she worked in her seriously underventilated studio.

This combination was bound to cause problems for the forty-six-year-old nonsmoker and she in fact did develop problems. First, came a chronic fever with flulike symptoms, followed by a tremor of her right hand during a two- to three-week period. Even when her energy level plummeted, she believed this "flu" would pass.

In the third week of her symptoms, Blair developed progressive low back pain and sciatica. Two years before, she'd had surgery for a herniated disk, which had gone well, so that wasn't the reason that her mood was flat and she had become depressed. As her cough and leg pain increased, she said to me, "I can't shake this flu. Could the paint I'm using be the cause of all these symptoms?"

Ultimately I requested a cadmium-level test, and when the results revealed a marked elevation of this mineral, I urged her to stop using the acrylic paints that contained it. She agreed to, and in two weeks her symptoms abated and her condition greatly improved.

The obvious lesson here is to be aware of the toxicities in seemingly innocent paints and crafts. There are other, equally vibrant paints available without cadmium's toxicity, but no matter which paint is chosen, using a mask and having proper ventilation is absolutely necessary while painting or using spray paints.

When many office workers complained often of general malaise and allergies, not specific illnesses, the term SBS gained a foothold. Before that, the mere thought of environmental toxins being emitted by a building was greatly derided, but by 1984, the World Health Organization was suggesting that up to 30 percent of new and remodeled buildings provided poor or hazardous air quality to the people who lived or worked in them.

Some of the factors contributing to SBS are:

- Biological contaminants (bacteria, molds, pollen, or viruses breed in stagnant water and accumulate in carpeting, ceiling tiles, ducts, and insulation).

- Chemical contaminants from carpeting, copy machines (ink chemicals), and cleaning agents.

- Inadequate ventilation.

- Outdoor chemical contaminants introduced by air conditioning, exhausts, and vents (bird droppings, which carry diseases communicable to humans, are often circulated through these systems).

Among the most widespread potential symptoms of sick building syndrome are brain fog, dizziness, eye and throat irritation, headache, nausea, poor concentration, or runny nose, as well as a general decrease in cognition. In many cases, these symptoms are relieved when the individual leaves the offending building.

Environmental forces, including toxins found in the workplace, are major factors in the increase of Alzheimer's, Parkinson's, and other brain diseases so prevalent today. Scientists are still discovering some of the long-term effects of sick building syndrome and, more important, how the highly toxic environment affects brain health.

Local and national regulations that mandated removing pollutants and improving ventilation and air-cleaning methods in large buildings have had a positive effect in reducing the number of SBS complaints. Unfortunately, many Americans still work in hazardous and unregulated environments.

Agricultural Toxins

Agricultural workers are especially susceptible to the effects of pesticides. A 1987 two-stage French study of 1,507 people sixty-five or older, with a five-year follow-up, revealed that farmers who had been exposed to pesticides or fungicides risked lower scores on the Mini-Mental Status examination, and that cognitive disturbance persists in occupationally exposed subjects long after they stop working. This study, reported in the *American Journal of Epidemiology* (March 1, 1993), also showed an increase in the risk for Parkinson's and Alzheimer's disease. Interestingly, the study reported the incidence of lowered cognitive ability even in people who lived near, but did not work in, the vineyards in this region of France.

INDUSTRIAL POLLUTANTS

Airport Toxins and Jet Fuel

When you are at the airport, noxious particles are continually circulating inside and outside the terminal—you are breathing in emissions while sitting at the gate, walking through the bridge, waiting for take off, or waiting for your bags. Although you may be unaware of the gaseous smell, which can be detected, you are taking in a combination of these toxins. In addition, the exhaust from burned jet fuel produces nitrous oxide, which depletes ozone and water vapor and has a negative impact on the climate. With all these potential dangers swirling about, I believe the airline industry should offer masks to travelers.

Diesel Fuel

Perhaps no method of transportation has been as demonized as the diesel engine, whose emissions continue to be a hazard. Many industries (and some drivers) prefer diesel fuel because of its lower cost and the durability of diesel engines, but the lower cost of operating diesel machinery comes at a very high price. Diesel fuel is a real threat to human health and the environment because diesel exhaust (whatever its source) contains more than forty known carcinogens. The manufacturers of diesel equipment are fully aware of this and, per an EPA mandate, they are currently modifying their products with an eye toward achieving a 70 percent reduction of hydrocarbon and carbon monoxide emissions in the next few years.

In addition, citizen groups and federal agencies have had a major impact on the reduction of diesel-fuel use. Especially rewarding to report is the recent settlement of the United States government against Toyota Motor Corporation for violation of the Clean Air Act. The case involved 2.2 million vehicles,

Fume Filters

Your car needs to have a filter for the outside air fumes when you drive— a standard feature in the newer cars. Be vigilant. As soon as you smell the fumes, apply a mask or wear a scarf or handkerchief to prevent breathing in these toxic fumes.

including many school buses manufactured between 1996 and 1998. In this prolonged courtroom drama, it was determined that the control systems of the offending vehicles had contributed measurably and irrefutably to ozone pollution. The health issues involved were an increase in asthma and other respiratory problems, and in some cases heart disease and compromised neurological systems in bus drivers, children, and pedestrians. Further, one of the chemicals found in the diesel-produced emissions is a known cofactor in strokes.

Pesticides

While manufacturers and, in tacit compliance, the United States government would have you believe that pesticides and insecticides are perfectly safe for humans, this is far from the truth. Both substances are highly neurotoxic. While there are some *pure* pesticides, which do affect only pests and vermin, most commercially used antipest products are insecticides that have the same effect on humans as on all other mammals.

They work by inhibiting the enzyme cholinesterase, which is essential for the transmission of nerve impulses, and neurotoxic symptoms of nausea, paralysis, tremors, weakness, and death can result. In the short term, the degree of these symptoms depends on the length of exposure. This, however, is just the beginning. These cholinesterase-inhibiting pesticides have been conclusively linked to major neurological problems in people. These are:

- Alzheimer's disease
- Chronic fatigue syndrome
- Parkinson's disease
- Pathological fetal development
- Slow cognitive development in children
- Stunted development in infants

DETERMINING YOUR LOCAL ENVIRONMENT'S TOXICITY QUOTIENT (TQ)

At this point you should understand why it is so important to take positive action against environmental toxins by learning what they are, where they come from, and how you can counterattack them. The larger question is what I call toxicity quotient (TQ). It is crucial to know what environmental toxins there are in your city, suburb, town, or rural area. For the sake of your health and your family's, you need to take an active role in learning the general TQ of your area in order to take informed action. The bad news is that chemicals are everywhere and in a much greater concentration than ever before.

In a perfect world, specifics would be available from your local city hall, chamber of commerce, the regional office of the EPA, or some other government arm, but if this is not an option, you can easily find information concerning the TQ of your area on the Internet at www.scorecard.org. You can type in your zip code at this extremely informative website and instantly obtain a list of all the known environmental toxins in your area. Samples of the information provided include the fact that in Chicago the risk level for cancer, including brain cancer, is more than 100 times greater than the risk level deemed acceptable by the Clean Air Act; Los Angeles is in the top 20 percent of all counties in the United States for toxins in the atmosphere; and the EPA has repeatedly cited the water supply of New York City as contaminated.

The website also has a list of the ten most toxic counties in the United States. As of this writing, they are:

1. Lee, Mississippi
2. Elkhart, Indiana
3. Harris, Texas
4. Erie, Pennsylvania
5. Logan, Kentucky
6. Monroe, New York
7. Georgetown, South Carolina
8. Gibson, Texas
9. Lazarus, Pennsylvania
10. Cook, Illinois

You will notice that, instead of the larger cities or metropolitan areas having the unhealthiest living environments, it's actually the smaller towns and rural areas. The reason is simple: These are where toxic waste plants and large manufacturing companies (including those that burn agricultural waste and chemicals) are most often located. This situation is not likely to change because in these remote, often economically depressed places, the residents are happy to have employment, and are therefore often unwilling to contest these companies' environmental practices. The reality is that their livelihood would be challenged.

I realize that being armed with information about the toxicity of your area is one thing, and acting on it is another. For most people, it's too difficult to pull up stakes, move a family, change a job, and start over. Nevertheless, I strongly urge you to find out as much as you can about the area in which you live, so you can make informed decisions based on the relative TQ of your area and change whatever can be changed in your environment. Being aware of toxic hazards may not only save your brain, but your life.

Concerning the manufacturers, the question is, should they be held responsible for the enormous health impacts of the *pesticide body burden*. I believe they should be, and I believe it is imperative that they truthfully inform the public whether or not a pesticide is harmful before distributing it for use. And the only way to ensure that information about a pesticide is made public is to become active and work toward instituting regulations mandating the release of such information.

IDENTIFYING YOUR ENVIRONMENTAL TOXICITIES

It is very difficult to avoid toxic substances in the environment, particularly those pollutants, such as insecticides, that you cannot see. It is also difficult to identify these problems because in today's world there is a daily barrage of auto exhaust, chemicals, chlorine gas, metals, phenols, and other environmental toxins in the air.

Do not lose hope. If you regularly experience such symptoms as flulike conditions, imbalance, a loss of circulation not traceable to a specific medical condition, or memory loss, you may be experiencing one or more reactions to pesticides or environmental toxins. The first step toward ameliorating the situation is to isolate the offending toxin, if possible.

If you visit a forward-thinking practitioner, he or she will question you about your lifestyle and your contact with potential toxic offenders, from mercury to lead to pesticides to exhaust and beyond. She or he will also try to determine lifestyle issues (*see* Chapter 10) that may be causing toxic-related symptoms and long-term neurological damage.

If you live in a metropolitan area, you should find an alternatively focused practitioner who will give these issues the respect and precision they deserve. If you believe you may be experiencing toxic reactions to your environment, the tools for detection include:

• Biochemical evaluation

• Blood analysis

• Special urinalysis tests to determine the body burden of toxic substances

Today, too many practicing physicians do not take the severity of environmental toxicity seriously enough, so you may have to initiate these tests yourself. (If you are forced to play a healthcare detective, the References section in back may be helpful.)

In the last decade there has been a wider realization that individuals themselves must take the lead in their personal health. No one can understand your physical, mental, and emotional needs better than yourself, and mainstream doctors seldom take the time anymore, anyway—those wonderful family doctors who took care of every detail of a family's health are a thing of the past. Today, with multiple diseases from soil depletion, environmental changes, the spread of diseases from other countries, even people's ignorance of personal hygiene, the world has changed, and so has medicine, which makes it important for people to think about their total health in a new multidimensional way.

Being aware and living every day as an informed individual really is paramount to your health. If you do nothing and think disease can only happen to the other guy or the person next door, you are wrong and you will indeed succumb to disease, so it is urgent to be diligent.

IS THERE A NONTOXIC FUTURE FOR PESTICIDES?

For too long, the pesticide industry has been in a holding pattern of overkill, but the tide is currently turning toward developing natural and less toxic products. The pressure is on as agriculture and an educated public have become driving forces for developing safer, friendlier products. Plant sources for organic or natural, nonchemical insecticides and pesticides are still largely untapped, but in the future plant-derived compounds may be the answer.

Synthetic pesticides have probably hit an impasse. Advances in biotechnology and chemistry are increasing the discovery and development of secondary compounds from plants. Environmental pressure is making a very strong and clear impact, and organic farming and agriculture is a dynamic force for our future.

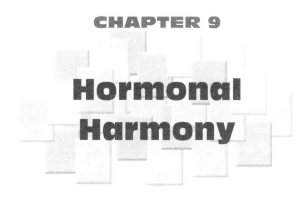

CHAPTER 9

Hormonal Harmony

Strong lives are motivated by dynamic purposes.
—Kenneth Hilderbrand

Hormones undergo a radical decline as people age. They peak at twenty years, stabilize for another decade, and then begin a steep decline. By the age of seventy, most people will have 50 percent fewer hormones than in their youth, a vital statistic because the importance of hormones in everyone's lives is irrefutable. Volumes of research continually show that declining hormones account for just about every negative aspect of aging—the decreased vision, the fragile bones, muscle loss, thinning skin, and the increased risk of depression, heart attacks, and strokes.

To reverse these effects, all hormones diminished by aging need to be replenished. The concept of replacing hormones has been an established medical practice for decades. Estrogen is the most widely prescribed drug in America, and I take my fellow physicians to task for stopping there. What is true for estrogen is true for all the other hormones.

Many physicians are uninformed about hormones. Most will treat only the symptoms until those symptoms manifest into disease, and will not think about prevention to deal with the inevitable fact that declining hormones will cause cellular disruption. Further, even physicians who do apply hormonal remedies do not administer the appropriate dosage. Some prescribe high, youthful levels of hormones. But because aging reduces the sensitivity of hormonal cell receptors, making them unresponsive to an overflow, flooding the body with large amounts of hormones is futile and sometimes damaging.

In this chapter, I will explain how hormonal replacement can slow down the aging process. It has taken three years to gather this up-to-the-minute information to help you create a personalized regimen. It will promote your overall brain health and your physical and mental longevity.

THE FUNCTIONS OF HORMONES

Hormones serve as molecular messengers. Governed by the brain, they regulate all the glands, which makes it imperative for brain health to be the focus of any anti-aging program. More than one hundred hormones influence the health of the body, and without the vital, influential brain hormones, it is not possible to enhance or retain memory. A prematurely aged brain will be useless in resisting the gradual decline of hormonal levels in the body.

Derived from Greek, the word hormone means *to set in motion.* These products of living cells circulate through the blood and can have an effect far from the site of origin. Hormones regulate who you are, and with all systems in the body modulated by hormonal regulation, hormonal balance is analogous to a symphony orchestra not missing a beat.

Hormonogenesis, the creation of hormones, is a process that is involved in every bodily function, and optimal health depends on the level of your hormones. These basic functions are: brain stimulation, blood pressure, body temperature, breathing, energy, fat burning, growth, heartbeat, immune system functioning, joint lubrication, memory process, and sleeping, plus the regulation of anxiety, depression, and stress. The endocrine glands, whether hypo or hyper, can be managed to bring our body and brain back into harmony. Your improved health is possible if you follow a hormonally supportive diet and supplement with vitamins, minerals, and bio-identical doses of natural hormone replacements.

The endocrine glands, which produce and release hormones into the bloodstream, are regulated to produce or not produce. When production doesn't meet bodily demand, the term hypo is added, as in *hypothyroidism.* If there is too much hormonal production, the term hyper is added, as in *hyperthyroidism.* Via the bloodstream, the hormones penetrate specific cells, acting on the genes within the cells' nuclei. Like a lock and key, the genetic code in the nucleus is unlocked, and it gives further access to information the cells require, including the signal to make more hormones if necessary.

THE FUNCTION OF BRAIN HORMONES

There are two kinds of brain hormones—those actually produced in the brain, and those that have a definitive effect on the brain. There are two very power-ful glands in the brain—the pituitary and the pineal—that influence the other glands by interaction with them, either stimulating or retarding production of the other hormones.

To repeat, hormones must be balanced. When a major hormone is insuf-ficient, it creates an imbalance and a synergistic effect develops, which can interrupt the effectiveness of the other hormones. The multihormonal approach for creating an appropriate balance is the safest and best chance for optimal health. To correct or replace a single hormone without knowing the status of additional important hormones is analogous to fixing just one flat tire when there are two. Hormone loss and imbalance is predictable with aging and is measured by testing. Function can be restored by supplementation. Pre-vention is a key here.

NATURAL HORMONES FOR THE BRAIN

Natural hormones refer to hormones produced by the body rather than those produced synthetically and added to the body. There are many vital natural hormones, but the ones discussed here have been chosen for their profound effect on the brain and memory. Although many are available over the counter, it is important to have baseline testing (blood or saliva) done before taking them in order to determine which, if any, hormones are depleted. Hor-mones are not innocuous. You are dealing with the master glands of the body, so professional guidance is mandatory in order to achieve the proper balance and not overdo—too much of a good thing can be very harmful.

Memory disorders are basically divided into three main categories: Age-associated mental impairment (AAMI); mild cognitive impairment (MCI); and dementia, including Alzheimer's disease. Their symptoms can be halted or reversed by replacing specific hormones that are deficient in the individual. Older people can often take as many as fifteen or twenty different medica-tions. In combination with decreased hormonal levels, this can cause severe dementia, which can be treated by reducing these medications and adding hormones via hormone replacement.

Dehydroepiandrosterone (DHEA)

DHEA, produced in the adrenal gland, skin, and brain, is a steroid hormone, as are estrogen and testosterone. Dr. William Regelson has called DHEA the "superstar of the super hormones" because of its effect on the body and the mind. Existing research has supported this hormone in its apparent ability to rejuvenate brain function and relieve the effects of stress. It is not without controversy, however, as some physicians believe DHEA may be harmful because of several negative side effects and discourage its use.

A dramatic drop in DHEA is often related to the development of arteriosclerosis, cancer, depression, and osteoporosis. As people get older, a deficiency in DHEA becomes more important since higher levels of the stress hormone cortisol appear, and DHEA, which can counter this, is less and less available to do so. If cortisol remains elevated for long periods, it can be toxic to brain cells, and this destructive process cannot be ignored.

Although DHEA insufficiency is common in both men and women, I have found in my practice that it is more prevalent in women. The beneficial antidepressant effect of DHEA is stronger in women, along with its positive increase in libido, improvement of skin tone, and possible protection from osteoporosis. There are women with adrenal hypofunction who desperately require DHEA replacement—in my practice, DHEA replacement in these women has resulted in less anxiety and a stronger libido. Physicians are more accepting of testosterone replacement for men, but they remain unaware of the need to replace DHEA. Its replacement can result in an increase of IgF-1 (a

DHEA Reverses Slowdown

I treated Margaret, a forty-five-year-old attorney who felt she was involuntarily slowing down because she had to read her briefs at least two or three times to understand and recall their content. She had lost her desire to go out at night with friends because she was always mentally and physically fatigued. In the morning, she had to drag herself out of bed, and just getting through her active day required a major effort. As her quality of life ebbed, her desperation increased. A hormone checkup revealed that her DHEA level was extremely low, and I prescribed a 25-mg dose of DHEA daily. This rewarded her with cognition, recall, and stamina. "In just one month I was back to normal," she said. "I looked and felt better, and I now have enough energy to complete an eighteen-hour day on my terms." In addition, Margaret's skin became softer, her hair glistened, and her feeling of well-being returned.

measure of growth hormone) and of total testosterone, which can improve erectile dysfunction in older men.

A negative effect of DHEA replacement includes a lowering of the HDL (good) cholesterol, which was reversed with pantothenic acid (vitamin B_5) or a slow nicotinamide supplement. Minor side effects, such as acne, facial-hair growth, and oily skin, were dose related and were diminished when the dose was reduced.

DHEA is converted by both sexes into estrogen and testosterone, producing more estrogen in women and more testosterone in men. DHEA peaks between ages twenty-five and thirty, then falls precipitously over time. At age eighty, DHEA is 10 to 15 percent of what it was at its peak.

Alzheimer's, Stress, and DHEA

In people with Alzheimer's disease, the DHEA level is low. The DHEA insufficiency in a neurotoxic degenerative process could impair the body's natural ability to repair and restore the damage inflicted on the brain. DHEA counters the effects of the stress hormone cortisol; if these effects are not countered, cortisol will produce damage, cell by cell.

Corticosteroids, such as cortisol, are damaging in older people because they remain in the system for longer periods of time than they do in younger people, thereby making the brain more vulnerable. Research papers show that when stress hormones are high, there is less ability to perform on memory tests. The cells within the hippocampus that are responsible for memory and learning are very susceptible to the presence of stress hormones. In people with Alzheimer's disease whose DHEA levels are low, I recommend supplementing with DHEA. Research in AIDS-related dementia has also shown a positive response to DHEA supplementation, since these people have a high level of stress hormones and low, if any, DHEA.

There is much speculation regarding the replacement of DHEA. The detractors believe there is still a lack of consensus about DHEA because, in animal studies, it raised cholesterol synthesis by 50 percent. Some negative studies presented in humans were dose related, meaning that the side effects such as facial hair growth did regress when the dose was lowered. The researchers see that in the lab this plentiful hormone defends the neuron from free radicals (an antioxidant function), enhances neuronal excitability, improves the neuronal plasticity (adaptation to experience), and plays a vital role in memory, but they do not know if it can do all that outside the lab.

New evidence reveals that DHEA can control the inflammatory response in some diseases, such as Alzheimer's. For every negative study, there are positive studies, although these are not always transferable to humans.

A major study of thousands of people is necessary, but it requires funding for a product that cannot be patented. It's the same old story—without a profit incentive, the drug companies are not the least bit motivated to engage in any DHEA studies on humans.

Anti-Aging and the DHEA Promise

In all the anti-aging programs I am aware of, DHEA is crucial. The ravages of aging can be modulated by replacing DHEA and other hormones and supplements that lab tests of blood, urine, saliva, etc. have shown to be low. These anti-aging programs require a change in lifestyle to help repair and renew bodily functions and reverse the downward spiral caused by the ravages of chronic illnesses.

The Immune Connection to DHEA

A weakened immune system accelerates the aging process and is responsible for the increase in cancer rates and for autoimmune diseases, such as rheumatoid arthritis. DHEA is an immune booster and can therefore help prevent traditional aging by fortifying the body against these chronic illnesses.

The immune system plays a complex role in defending the body through immunotransmitters known as cytokines. These natural proteins have the ability to relay messages between components, and can mount an immune response to many biological challenges. The three types of cytokines are interleukins, tumor necrosis factor (TNF), and interferons, and they all mobilize against any threatened invasion by coordinating the white-cell response to infection and injury.

Cytokines are the e-mail of the immune system. They deliver a warning to speed up or slow down the immune system's response to a threat of invasion. Cytokine interleukin-1 promotes sleep and curtails appetite.

The downside of cytokines is that they can cause depression, fatigue, and impaired thinking. The gamma interferon cytokine can inhibit the brain's ability to produce serotonin, which causes depression. Interleukin is partly responsible for the production of beta-amyloid, which can kill brain cells and destroy memory. Interleukin cytokines are implicated in apoptosis (programmed cell death), and it is postulated that Alzheimer's disease and Parkinson's disease may be a result of apoptosis, perhaps mediated through specific cytokines.

The pathway to success in restoring the immune system may be in the neutralizing effect of DHEA on stress hormones, which can reduce the immune system's effectiveness. By neutralizing these stress hormones, DHEA can bolster the immune system's function.

In a University of Wisconsin study, Dr. Omid Khoram linked the importance of DHEA to immune function. He studied the immune systems of nine healthy older men who took DHEA for five months and found that DHEA was able to rejuvenate the aging immune system in these men. The studies revealed that the immune-enhancer IgF-1 was elevated and that IL-6 cytokine linked to autoimmune disease was normalized. Further, cytokine IL-2, responsible for boosting the immune system, was increased, B-cell production was stimulated, and NK (natural killer) cancer-fighting cells were also increased.

The studies of Dr. Regelson and Dr. Kalimi demonstrate the protective effect of DHEA against stress hormones, which, if unopposed, can cause havoc with the immune system and have a major negative impact on the brain.

The Memory-Restoration Connection

Complaints about memory usually start in the forties or fifties and increase with age. People who supplement with DHEA often say their memory is improved and their thinking is more focused.

The initial human trials of DHEA for memory took place in the 1980s. At the City of Hope Hospital in Duarte, California, studies utilized DHEA's effect on brain function. The scientists took tissue cultures of brain cells and placed them in a petri dish to grow, adding the DHEA. The DHEA stimulated the growth of axons and dendrites, thus aiding in the growth of brain networks by forming interconnections.

A second study at this hospital utilized young and old mice in a maze experiment. If a mouse went in the wrong direction, he received a small electrical shock. Young mice quickly learned to avoid the shock and proceed in the correct direction. Older mice did not perform as well except when they were given an injection of DHEA, following which they also breezed through the maze. Two weeks after all the older mice were tested, those with DHEA retained the memory of the maze pattern, as did the younger mice.

Can this result apply to humans? There have been positive studies indicating the value of DHEA for memory in humans. In a basic study conducted by Dr. Owen Wolkowitz from the Department of Psychiatry at the University of California, San Francisco, six depressed, middle-aged men with memory impairment were given 60–90 mg of DHEA for four to six weeks. All the men showed improvement in both depression and memory, and their ability to recall markedly improved.

Dr. Wolkowitz is directing studies fostered by the National Institute on Aging to determine the value of DHEA for people with Alzheimer's disease, and psychological testing will show if the addition of DHEA has improved the quality of life for these people. Other studies have shown that higher doses are not necessarily effective. Youthful levels should be sufficient because the brain can be overwhelmed by high doses and overloading can occur. Dosage compatible with what is naturally produced by the body may be all that is necessary.

The Estrogen Conundrum

Combined hormone therapy (estrogen plus progesterone) has been a mainstay for many years, with virtually thousands of scientific papers supporting its protective effects for Alzheimer's disease, dementia, heart disease, and strokes. The support has been ongoing for estrogen's protective effects on the brain—improving blood flow, reducing cholesterol, reducing neuronal loss, and modulating the AD gene (APO-lipoprotein E).

However, a major trial of combined hormone therapy, the Women's Health Initiative study, was discontinued after five and a half years instead of its planned eight and a half years because the findings pointed to an increased risk of breast cancer, heart disease, pulmonary embolism, and strokes, which outweighed any beneficial effects of estrogen and progesterone. Published in *The Journal of the American Medical Association* (*JAMA*), this was the largest study ever done, and its conclusion left many women in a quandary as to what to do. The uproar was partially fueled by the press, which had a field day, often misstating the study and its results.

The conclusion read in part, "Despite the significant negative effect of estrogen plus progestin on the risk for developing probable dementia, our findings need to be kept in perspective. Although participants assigned to active therapy are at twice the risk for dementia, the absolute risk is relatively small. . . . Moreover, while most women did not experience a negative treatment effect on cognition, a small increased risk of clinically meaningful cognitive decline occurred in the estrogen plus progestin group." My interpretation is that the number of patients affected was not enough to significantly discontinue the use of HRT without further selectivity and lower-dose consideration.

Is this much ado about nothing? The study was restricted to women age sixty-five or more, much older than the typical HRT users, and who were using the drug to treat menopausal symptoms. Also, the results were based on synthetic equine estrogen and medroxyprogesterone acetate. According to a subsequent 2003 *JAMA* article, this study resulted in a diminished use of HRT with estrogen and progesterone because of their side effects. The next follow-up study will be released in 2010.

In the study, 16,608 postmenopausal women had a 31 percent increase of total stroke risk compared to the placebo group after one year of treatment with the equine estrogen plus progestin. But I have to ask, what if women had used natural estrogen or phytoestrogen? What if they had taken a baby aspirin daily to lessen thrombosis? Neither of these issues were addressed in the studies.

The study demonstrated a 26 percent increase in breast cancer in the third year when estrogen and progesterone were prescribed. Combined menopausal hormone therapy reveals a diminished sensitivity to mammograms because of increased tissue density in the breast, and the estrogen plus progesterone has been shown to cause a proliferation of normal breast tissue and may conceal breast cancer. Although this did not occur in the majority of subjects tested, it is of concern in those who have developed such a density, which may conceal a lesion.

I believe the problem is actually with the interpretation of these studies and the fact that the type of estrogen in this study was derived from mare's urine. Progestin is also a synthetic. Dr. Elizabeth Vliet, who has written three books about women and hormones, believes that estrogen from a mare's urine is inferior because it does not contain estradiol, a different form of estrogen. The current hormonal replacement therapies (HRT) do use estradiol, which is identical to the estrogen produced in the body during a woman's reproductive years. Natural progesterone was not studied as thoroughly and received little or no press. These newer forms of replacement therapy may have fewer side effects than the synthetic hormones. One alternative plant-derived estrogen and progesterone is Activella, and there are other hormonal alternatives. Compounding pharmacies are equipped to make, by prescription, natural hormone combinations that were not part of this condemning study.

Hot Flashes

The primary reason women request medical attention for menopausal symptoms are hot flashes, which can persist for five to fifteen years following the first signs of menopause, the perimenopausal period. Waking up drenched in sweat is draining, and the loss of sleep is intolerable. Seventy-five percent of women experience hot flashes, and the heat and sweat sensations are often accompanied by anxiety, irritability, even palpitations. The exact reason for this disturbance is still unknown, but it is believed that the normal thermoregulatory system has gone awry.

Some studies suggest that SSRI antidepressants (selective serotonin reuptake inhibitors) may reduce the vasomotor (constriction or dilation of blood vessels) symptoms associated with hot flashes. According to the June 2003 *JAMA* article mentioned on page 165, Dr. Vered Stearns found that paroxetine CR (Paxil) relieved hot flashes in a general population of menopausal women after six weeks of therapy. The study provided new and valuable information on the treatment of hot flashes and also provided an alternative to HRT.

Many gynecologists stopped renewing prescriptions for HRT (equine), but offered no alternative treatment. Clearly these women are unhappy with their resurgence of sweats day and night. So far, my female patients who come in for hormonal problems or neurological complaints, tell me they would not discontinue HRT "no matter what." Most of these women were on combina-

Natural Alternatives Restore Balance

Katherine is fifty-six years old and had her last period four months prior to seeing me. She had ongoing menopausal symptoms, which included hot flashes, sleepless nights, vaginal dryness, and brain fog every morning. I recommended a reduced carbohydrate diet, an increase of protein and fresh vegetables, and high-potency vitamins. Additional lab tests showed that she had a low zinc level and an elevated homocysteine level, so I added B_6, B_{12}, folic acid, and zinc to her regimen.

A hormonal blood panel showed which hormones required supplementation. She responded well to bio-identical estrogen and micronized natural progesterone. I added DHEA, pregnenolone, and testosterone to a formulated transdermal cream which she applied in the morning and evening. Six weeks later, Katherine was a happy woman—the hot flashes were infrequent and her sleeping patterns and energy levels were much improved. She is still energetic, her hormones are in sync, and she is pleased to be back in balance.

tion therapy, utilizing equine estrogen and unnatural progesterone until I switched them to a natural, low-dose product, thereby reducing risk. My advice is to find a practitioner who will work with you and help you find alternatives.

My Perspective

In the last two years, the mainstream media only wrote about major HRT studies on synthetic hormones (Premarin and Prempro). The alternative, bio-identical hormones were never discussed and this vital omission has caused women unnecessary problems.

As noted, the women studied were on HRT *after* menopause, but the more common therapeutic use of HRT is for symptoms connected with the *onset* of menopause, the perimenopausal period. I have to wonder what the results would have been if the study had focused on perimenopausal women. A reevaluation of some of the women in the study who were on HRT may have shown they did not require hormone therapy. For women who do require HRT, bio-identical hormones will be the answer. Compounding pharmacies can fill your doctor's prescription to fit your exact needs. Switching from Premarin or Prempro to a natural (plant-based) form of estrogen and progesterone will require a transitional period of two to four months. Remember that exercise, nutritional support, and stress reduction are essential for a successful health program for women (and men).

Growth Hormone (Somatotropin)

Growth hormone (GH) remains the most controversial hormone. Every week my office will receive a call specifically for a GH prescription. The callers are not interested in a full evaluation to determine the need for supplementation—they simply wish to find the fountain of youth at any physical or mental cost.

Is this hormone all hype? Is it merely a substitute for lack of exercise, diet awareness, and a healthy lifestyle? In my opinion, whatever beneficial effects GH may have can be achieved by balancing other super hormones, in particular DHEA, estrogen, melatonin, and testosterone. GH should be reserved for special extreme circumstances, such as the death of heart muscle, helping to restore a failing organ or reverse severe osteoporosis or renal failure. There is no question that growth hormone is important as people age. There is a dramatic decline of GH in each decade—its decline is inevitable. Further, severe illness and the stress of living can interfere and reduce the body's production of this hormone. Peak production of growth hormone comes in the teenage years, with spurts throughout adolescence. Although GH is important for growth, growing taller is only part of the beneficial picture. GH also decreases body fat, promotes lean body mass and muscle growth, and enhances bone strength. Research has shown that supplementing with this hormone enhances mood and a sense of well-being.

The master gland, the pituitary, makes growth hormone. It is found deep in the brain, well protected from most trauma. The level of GH in the blood changes throughout the day, but its peak production occurs during sleep. By restoring testosterone in men and estrogen in women to youthful levels, we can enhance the production of GH—a major reason initially for not needing to prescribe injections of GH.

Growth hormone is related to a hormone known as IgF-1 (insulin-like growth factor) produced by the liver. DHEA increases the production of IgF-1. The synergy of these DHEA and GH hormones is remarkable. Children who do not have enough growth hormone are dwarfed, and their life expectancy is lowered. In older adults, there can be a malfunction of the pituitary gland, characterized by depression, elevated cholesterol, loss of libido, a loss of muscle strength, osteoporosis (more than usual), a weakened immune system, and sleep disturbances—all similar to aging. When GH was given to older adults who were hormone deficient due to this malfunction, these symptoms were reversed.

In 1990, excitement reigned when Dr. Daniel Rudman of the Medical College of Wisconsin published a research paper in *The New England Journal of Medicine*. The study concerned twenty-one healthy men from ages sixty-one to eighty-one who all had low levels of IgF-1. Twelve of these men received GH injections three times a week for six months. The remaining nine men served as controls in the study and were not treated. Those taking the injections of

Caveat

You should be aware that negative side effects of GH supplementation include carpal tunnel syndrome, diabetes, joint pains, swollen breasts in males, and a possible risk of prostate cancer, not to mention that noses and limbs can grow disproportionately to the face and body. Further, its positive effect on the brain is inconclusive. At the University of California, San Francisco, endocrinologist Maxine Papadakis treated older men with growth hormone for six months, and the results revealed a mild improvement on tests of attention, but a slight decrease in cognition.

GH increased physically in all parameters, including bone density. Dr. Rudman concluded that those who received six months of GH experienced a reversal equivalent to ten to twenty years of changes. These historical findings renewed interest in the possible slowing of the aging process.

Studies sponsored by The National Institute on Aging and others continue to determine whether GH can be an aid in keeping older people vigorous and strong. Some studies have been negative due to the side effects. Still other studies failed to show a demonstrably positive effect on mood or an increase in cognition.

The loss of muscle in older people is inevitable since stem cells in the bone marrow, which replace muscle tissue, cannot keep up the pace of the demands of daily living, and no study has convincingly shown that GH is more effective than vigorous exercise. The abuse of GH by bodybuilders may significantly decimate hormonal balance later in their lives.

On a positive note, the experience of Dr. Chein in Palm Springs, California, has been very pro-GH for its "ability to reverse biological aging." He has treated more than 1,000 people and confirms that "fat decreases, muscle mass increases, lung capacity improves, heart function is better, bone density increases and skin thickens." He also claims that the immune system improves, as demonstrated by an increase in antibody production and restored NK (natural killer) cell activity.

In her 2003 article published in *The New England Journal of Medicine,* Dr. Mary Lee Vance reviewed the Rudman study and other larger studies. There are three areas of concern. First, in older people, resistance exercise significantly increased muscle strength, and the addition of GH did not result in further improvement. Second, she voices concerns over long-term GH administration because it may be harmful to older people. There is concern about a risk for cancer since GH increases serum concentrations of IgF-1. The evidence supporting the association of elevated IgF-1 (a measure for active GH in your body) and cancer is mounting, yet there is no clear link to a cause. If you already have cancer, GH may enhance the growth of cancer cells. Third, she is concerned about the misuse of healthcare resources. One-third of the prescriptions for GH are off-label and not approved by the FDA.

Additional studies post-1990 have not confirmed the effect of GH in improving function. "There is no current magic bullet that retards or reverses aging," Dr. Vance said, "Anti-aging with GH has not yet been proved effective according to objective outcome criteria." Adding to that argument, the National Institutes of Health reported that none of the over-the-counter GH supplements have prevented or reversed aging. Dr. Chein has cautioned patients about the risk of taking hormone supplements purchased over the counter. "They are not pharmaceutical grade," he said, "and may be impure, not natural, not of the specific potency claimed—they are risky."

The controversy continues. My suggestion is to balance all the other hormones first and then consider GH, being aware of the possible side effects.

Amino Acid Stackers

There is speculation that young people may benefit from taking multiple amino acids together on an empty stomach. These releasers—arginine, glutamine, lysine, and ornithine—so called because they may help release more GH (growth hormone) and IgF-1 from this synergistic effect. At this time, there is no science to support this.

Insulin

Insulin is a protein hormone synthesized in the pancreas and secreted by clumps of cells within the pancreas that make it and other hormones. Insulin is essential for the metabolism of carbohydrates, fats, and proteins.

Sometimes with no obvious symptoms, insulin may be attacking your arteries, increasing your blood pressure, and causing fatigue. Although vital to life in normal quantities, it can be pernicious, or even lethal, in excess. The neutralization of excess insulin is critical since it is a cause of diabetes, heart disease, and strokes. Over time, as you gain weight, insulin levels can rise along with your glucose, and this can increase your cholesterol and triglycerides.

The Impact of Insulin on the Brain

Besides feeding glucose to cell tissues and muscles, insulin is vital to brain cells. Studies beginning in the mid-1980s found receptors for insulin within the brain, and supplements of insulin-enhancing agents were found to improve memory in animals, which suggests that insulin may be protective to brain cells and memory.

Another study has shown that insulin can prevent the formation of tangles (abnormal proteins) within the brain. In a study of college students who had slightly abnormal insulin functioning, the results demonstrated a lower level of performance—poor recollection of a list of words—which suggested that the insulin system is involved in the memory process. Not all questions concerning insulin can be answered by research at this time, but studies in genetic and molecular medicine are expected to soon provide additional answers regarding the brain.

Receptors for insulin have been found in the hippocampus, a part of the limbic system that plays a role in converting new information into long-term memory, and the hypothalamus, a deep part of both sides of the brain and a regulatory center for food control.

Insulin and Diabetes

The primary ability of this hormone is to facilitate the uptake of glucose into the cells of the body and regulate the release of glucose from the liver; its primary purpose is to control blood-sugar levels and prevent diabetes. This is critical, and when the pancreatic cells are in sync, insulin can help protect blood vessels, strengthen the immune and digestive systems, create energy reserves, store fat, and increase endurance.

In type I diabetes, the lack of insulin (when the pancreas fails to make sufficient insulin) can manifest as juvenile diabetes, or diabetes at any age. When insulin production doesn't meet the intake of glucose, the result can be diabetes.

In type II (insulin resistance) diabetes there is excess insulin in the blood, and it has become ineffective in lowering the high glucose. The term *insulin resistance* was first coined by Gerald Reaven, M.D., Emeritus Professor of Medicine from the Stanford School of Medicine. A recent study at this university emphasized the need for heart and brain protection in people with type II diabetes since there is risk to both organs because excess insulin damages blood vessels. Additional research at Stanford noted the risk of inflammation linked to insulin resistance, which causes the smooth muscle cells in the vessels to proliferate with a propensity to clog or obstruct the flow in the vessels. The drug researched in this study is rosiglitazone (Avandia). One of the study's researchers, Dr. James Chu, stated, "Because more people with diabetes die of heart disease, a drug that potentially can treat multiple facets of the insulin-resistance syndrome is exciting."

At this time, type II diabetes is occurring in epidemic proportions, impacting 25 percent of the American population. It is most common in obese individuals. A diet overabundant in sugar and carbohydrates leads to increased insulin levels, which, in turn, causes the body to store more fat. A sugar imbalance, particularly an up-and-down, yo-yo effect, can result in poor concentration and memory deficits. There can also be an increased vulnerability to depression since high insulin decreases serotonin levels, causing anxiety, depression, and mood changes.

The brain, the body's master control system, weighs only about three pounds. This is probably less than 2 percent of the body's weight, yet it uses 20 percent of the oxygen and 50 percent of the energy supply to feed its brain cells (there are more than a billion of these neurons).

Healthy, diabetes-free people have less than a teaspoonful of sugar in their blood. How much do you have? What should you do if you have more sugar than normal? I suggest switching to a diet of complex carbohydrates, including grains, legumes, vegetables, and nuts, all of which are basically time-released and do not require a larger shot of insulin to enter the system.

The Insulin Link to Alzheimer's Disease

There have been studies on Alzheimer's disease to ascertain whether a low level of insulin in the brain has much to do with a primary memory disorder. Many people with Alzheimer's have low levels of insulin in their spinal fluid, suggesting there could be a problem in processing this hormone.

The June 2003 *Journal of Neurology* reported a study by Dr. Suzanne Craft at the VA Puget Sound Health Care System in Seattle, Washington, which suggests that high levels of insulin can boost the production of brain proteins linked to Alzheimer's disease. This small, speculative study revealed that giving older people high doses of insulin increased the amount of protein that forms plaques in the brains of people with Alzheimer's disease, suggesting that lowered insulin levels could delay or prevent Alzheimer's disease. The results emphasized the importance of treating and preventing diabetes. "High insulin levels are bad for your brain as well as your body," said Dr. Craft.

The Insulin-Aging Connection

Aging is augmented by elevated insulin. An overgrowth of smooth muscle cells in the arterial wall causes hardening of the arteries, and the result is less and less blood flow until the vessel cuts the flow off altogether and a heart attack or stroke occurs. Insulin also has a negative effect on the body's plaque-dissolving system, again promoting plasminogen activator inhibitor-1, which, when elevated, reduces its fibrinolytic action, encouraging an increased risk for arterial and venous thrombosis (clot formation).

Cholesterol production is increased by insulin liver stimulation. LDL (dense LDL particles) becomes oxidized, also as a result of increased insulin, and contributes to a major vessel obstruction. Triglyceride elevation is stimulated by the elevation of insulin as well, and the good HDL cholesterol falls when it is needed most. Hypertension is also related to insulin resistance, and its elevation is due to the vasoconstriction of the blood vessels. Lastly, in the laboratory, insulin has stimulated malignant cells.

How to Control the Insulin-Aging Connection

- Drink alcohol only in moderation, not excessively. According to Dr. Reaven's studies at Stanford, one to two alcoholic drinks daily had the effect of lowering blood sugar as well as insulin. It also promoted a higher HDL (good cholesterol) level.

- Eat less at one sitting, as blood sugar and insulin become elevated following a big meal. I encourage six small meals a day.

- Eliminate polyunsaturated fats. Corn and sunflower oils that oxidize faster, increasing glucose and releasing insulin, can create more free radicals. You must have enough antioxidants to offset this barrage of free radicals.

- Include healthy monosaturated fats in your diet, such as those found in avocados, nuts, olives, and canola oil. These fats prolong oxidation and do not cause a rush of insulin around a cascade of glucose.

- Lose weight. Obesity suppresses insulin's ability to process glucose. You can often reverse an insulin problem by losing weight.

- Reduce carbohydrates. Create a plan with a certified nutritionist or a nutritionally aware healthcare practitioner.

- Take chromium. 200 mcg of organic chromium makes insulin more efficient and helps keep it down.

- Take antioxidant vitamin E. It protects the cell membranes from free-radical damage, thereby helping cells use insulin more effectively to transport glucose. I suggest 400–800 IU a day.

Melatonin

The pineal gland is a pebble-sized structure deep within the brain that releases melatonin, the hormone referred to by Hindu mystics and yogis as the third eye. The release of this hormone regulates the body's sleeping and waking cycle, makes you aware of environmental changes, and enables night and day adaptation. The sensitivity of the pineal gland cells is ignited by light entering the eye through the pupil, focusing on the retina. The path is through the optic nerve to the cells in the hypothalamus, a regulatory center. The relay to the pineal gland indicates light or dark and determines the amount of melatonin produced. The dark stimulates production, whereas light will suppress it.

Melatonin helps maintain homeostasis (balance), indirectly affecting the other hormones. In the mid-forties or earlier, melatonin begins a steep decline because the pineal gland cells begin to shrink. At ages sixty to seventy, the body produces less than half of the melatonin of earlier times.

In *The Superhormone Promise,* Dr. William Regelson says that melatonin does not just treat the causes of aging at the surface, but it goes to a much deeper root level. "Melatonin alters the very environment that allows the aging process to take hold," he writes. Also, melatonin inhibits the harmful effects of stress hormones and helps prevent autoimmune diseases. Melatonin can also enhance endorphins, the stress-relieving chemicals produced by the immune system and the brain, and thereby helps to withstand the stresses of illness. Free-radical damage is thwarted by melatonin, an antioxidant, and keeping a normal melatonin level can help avoid plaque formation in the blood-vessel wall that could result in a subsequent heart attack or stroke.

Animal studies indicate melatonin may be of value in life extension—older mice supplemented with melatonin lived 25 percent longer than the other mice. Humans have not been tested.

1–3 mg at bedtime may be helpful.

Note: Anyone with an autoimmune disease, epilepsy, renal disease, or severe allergies should not take melatonin.

Pregnenolone (PREG)

Sometimes called the parent of the sex hormones, pregnenolone is a super hormone produced by the brain and adrenal cortex from which DHEA is derived. Pregnenolone's production decreases with age, and at seventy-five only 30 to 40 percent of youthful levels is produced. The production of PREG in the body comes through cholesterol, which is ingested in foods and made by the liver.

Pregnenolone is a safe, nontoxic element of a life-extension program. Studies have shown that it facilitates learning as a memory enhancer. It can also reduce stress and increase well-being. At youthful levels, concentration and psychomotor performance are improved. Some common medicinal plants, such as wild yam, contain diosgenin, which chemically converts to pregnenolone. There is a synergistic effect between the hormones DHEA and melatonin. This combination can reduce cravings for alcohol, caffeine, and nicotine.

Typically for a natural substance, even a hormone, there is no profit motivation for the drug companies to promote pregnenolone. When research on PREG had just begun in the 1940s, pregnenolone was put aside as researchers switched to cortisone, a closely related hormone, because corticosteroids could be patented. And with patents came the ability to charge more. As the harmful side effects of corticosteroids came into sharper focus, so did a renewed interest in PREG research, beginning again in 1996.

Steroids resemble each other in that they all have a four-carbon ring structure. As with pregnenolone, cortisol, DHEA, estrogen, progesterone, and testosterone are all steroid hormones, differing only in small structural changes. PREG is produced in the adrenal gland and brain, as well as in other organs. The brain converts cholesterol into pregnenolone and other steroids. PREG converts to DHEA, which in turn converts into estrogens, androgens, and other steroids. PREG can form the other hormones, such as progesterone, and it is one of the steroids that is produced in the mitochondria of the eye's retinal cells.

Eugene Roberts, Ph.D., of the neurobiochemistry department at the City of Hope/Beckman Research Institute, Duarte, California, has stated that PREG "appears to be the most potent memory enhancer in animals." Research in humans is still forthcoming. As with all hormones, do not take pregnenolone without consulting a healthcare practitioner knowledgeable in hormone usage.

The Thyroid Hormones

The thyroid gland is located in the front of the throat at the base of the neck. It secretes the hormones thyroxine (T-4), which is 90 percent of its output, and the most active hormone, triiodothyronine (T-3), which is about 10 percent. The pituitary gland, located in the mid-interior of the brain between the two hemispheres, releases the thyroid-stimulating hormone (TSH), which stimulates the thyroid gland to release its two hormones.

The thyroid gland is of major importance because of its overall effect on the body and, specifically, its profound influence on the brain. Thyroid hormones speed metabolism and help control weight. They boost circulation in the blood and keep the skin soft and warm, and they make joints and muscles more pliable, probably due to an increase in blood flow. A balanced thyroid improves the flow of blood to the brain and is extremely vital to memory and concentration. Fatigue, sensitivity to cold, and sluggish thinking relates to a poorly functioning thyroid gland, as do hair loss, puffiness of the face, and swollen eyelids.

Thyroid hormones have an effect on all the body's systems, including arteries, cholesterol distribution, fat-burning, the heart, and the immune system. Undiagnosed hyperthyroidism can lead to heart disease, strokes, and other health problems, and constipation, particularly in older people and those with Parkinson's, results from a dysfunction of the powerful thyroid gland.

In my active practice, I find that some of my patients have thyroid disease that went unnoticed by other doctors they had visited. For the physician, the key here is to always do more than rely on laboratory data, particularly when it involves hypothyroidism. The practitioner has to listen very carefully for such words as *fatigue, tired, depressed,* or *no energy,* which are often indicative of hypothyroidism. Some of my patients ask, "Since I eat very little and I exercise, why am I gaining weight?" and I have to tell them that bloating and weight gain can also be a sign of hypothyroidism.

Thyroid Self-Testing

It is significant to note that blood tests indicating so-called *normal* thyroid function can be as much as 30 percent inaccurate, and they often miss hypothyroidism. You can easily test your own thyroid activity with the self-testing thyroid-temperature test, which is generally accurate.

More than fifty years ago, Dr. Broda Barnes suggested that the body's basal temperature was an accurate indicator of thyroid activity. Taking your axillary (under the arm) temperature when you first wake up and before you get out of bed will measure your basal metabolic rate. This indicates thyroid activity. The less the activity, the more accurate the results.

Here's how it works: Upon awakening, while still lying down, place a digital thermometer inside your axilla (armpit). Record the temperature reading, the time, and the date (after it beeps). The result is your A.M. basal temperature, normally between 97.8 and 98.2. Even if lab results say the thyroid is in normal range, your thyroid output is low if your temperature remains below 97.8 for at least four days. (Menstruating women should not do these temperatures during their period, as the results will be askew.) If your thyroid results are out of range, you may want to discuss them with an alternatively oriented healthcare practitioner who can prescribe the appropriate amount of natural thyroid and follow up with you. It will make a tremendous difference.

Prevalence of Thyroid Problems

Thyroid disease affects 20 million Americans each year, and women are ten times more prone to thyroid dysfunction than men. In addition, six months after giving birth, 5 percent of women develop a thyroid disorder. This is because during pregnancy women's immune response to disease is suppressed,

Fatigue and Fainting Are Banished

Jim is a forty-six-year-old electrical engineer and researcher for a major corporation. He came to me for occasional episodes of lightheadedness and syncope (fainting that results from insufficient blood flow to the brain). His history was unremarkable until the past three years when he felt overwhelming fatigue and a gradual loss of his spontaneous and creative self. His lethargy began when he woke up in the morning and was more severe by 4 P.M. His hair became thinner, and his libido was nil.

To me, Jim was the typical thyroid-deficient patient. Since two diagnoses can coexist, I requested a magnetic resonance angiogram (MRA) to be sure that his carotid arteries were clear and that vascular disease was not a cause of his syncope. The study showed he was fine on that score, but his blood work indicated a probable low thyroid. To confirm this, I requested he take his temperature daily for five days, and when it did not measure above 96.5 five mornings in a row, I knew he had a low-functioning thyroid gland. Per my prescription, he began taking 60 mg of Armour (natural) thyroid, and ten days later, this six-foot-two-inch patient came in all aglow. "I could hug and kiss you," he said. "I am back to my old self. It's like coming out of a dark room into the light."

I was not the first doctor to test Jim for hypothyroidism, but it had not registered in his previous thyroid tests with other doctors. All his prior blood work had been normal. I have often found that the blood work is correct only 80 percent of the time, whereas the body temperature used in the Barnes method is very accurate and will support the diagnosis.

and following delivery a rebound of the immune system can cause an inflammation of the thyroid gland. Postpartum thyroid dysfunction is frequently missed because the symptoms are blamed on postpartum depression, but in a new mother, a low-functioning thyroid gland (hypothyroidism) can cause prolonged depression, lethargy, a decrease in cognition, and loss of libido. It is important to treat this in order to prevent numerous complications and enhance the new mother's quality of life.

Memory, Dementia, and the Thyroid

Memory loss or dementia related to a poorly functioning thyroid gland should not be difficult to diagnose. (Memory loss is a symptom of dementia, which is persistent and often progressive, but normal forgetfulness probably does not interfere with everyday life in a dramatic way.) The gland is under instructions from the pituitary, the master gland in the brain, which releases thyroid-stimulating hormone (TSH) that controls how much thyroid hormone is to be released into the bloodstream to regulate the body's metabolism. Neither immediate recall nor past recall are age dependent, and until it is recognized and treated, a poorly functioning thyroid gland can affect both.

Retirement Blues Retired

Madeline is a fifty-two-year-old designer who was extremely successful as a CEO of her own design business for twenty-five years. When she came to see me, both she and her husband had just retired and were about to take a postretirement vacation. Madeline said she had been sleeping poorly for approximately six to eight weeks and that she felt anxious, as though she was going into a downward spiral of uneasiness and depression. According to her husband, she was displaying bouts of irritability and was not herself. She thought menopause was a cause of the problems, or that she was sad about handing over control of her business to someone else. Following their return from vacation, her nervousness and anxiety increased, and her husband insisted she get tested. When the blood tests revealed that her thyroid gland was too active (hyperthyroidism), I was able to reduce the overactivity by using radioactive iodine. It shrank the gland in a few weeks, and Madeline was finally able to enjoy her well-earned retirement.

Back Pain Backs Off

I examined Benjamin, a fifty-three-year-old corporate executive, for painful arthritis symptoms in his back (arthritis can be associated with hypothyroidism). Having to sit during prolonged meetings added to his low-back syndrome. The back pain was caused by inflammation of some of the joints in his lower back, and he was taking various anti-arthritis medications, which gave him only short, incomplete relief. After I had taken a careful history, he admitted to never feeling fresh when he woke up and to being so fatigued by 4 P.M. that he often fell asleep at his desk.

Following my instructions on how to use the Broda Barnes method, he recorded five days of low temperatures, which indicated that he needed thyroid replacement, although his blood work again showed he was borderline for low thyroid. After putting him on a moderate thyroid replacement program for two weeks, his energy levels rose, and he required lower and lower doses of anti-inflammatory medication for his receding back pain. He can now tolerate more exercise, and sitting through long business meetings is no longer the torture for him that it once was.

The immune system, particularly in women, can develop antibodies that attack the thyroid gland, causing Hashimoto's thyroiditis. This can cause either a hypo or hyper function of the thyroid gland, and either level has an effect on brain function. Although some studies suggest that hypothyroidism may increase the frequency of Alzheimer's disease, thyroid disease has not usually been suspected, particularly in relation to older people. In order to save brain function, a closer investigation of thyroid function needs to be routine.

Neurotransmitters (NT)

Neurotransmitters are chemicals that transmit nerve impulses across a synapse. They are in this chapter because they are included in the hormone family, although they differ in the location of their action. Hormones travel from their gland of origin through the blood to a point of action some distance from their formation, but neurotransmitters are formed at the synapse (junction), the gap between nerve structures where the nerve impulse passes from one neuron to another, and have almost no need to travel since their action is within that synapse. Neurotransmitters such as dopamine, norepinephrine, and serotonin all have a role in managing hormone function. The composition of all hormones is closely related to neurotransmitters and influences the amount and reaction of neurotransmitters released in the brain. There are well more than a hundred neurotransmitters working in your body and brain at any given time, and since almost all of them play a role in memory, their importance cannot be underestimated.

Neuron action is analogous to how a computer receives and processes messages, which are then sent to another computer. The neuron's message is a chemical one, which interacts with the outer surface of a cell membrane. This chemical interaction creates a chemical change within the receiving neuron, and the constant exchange of chemical messages is known as neurotransmission. Neurons release specific neurotransmitters via polarization, depolarization, action potentials, electrolyte changes, and the firing of an electrical impulse.

The neurotransmitters float across the synapse until they meet with the dendrite, which carries messages toward the cell body of the next neuron. On the dendrite are specific receptors to which neurotransmitters bind. The sending neuron is the original neuron. The neuron that binds the neurotransmitter is the receiving neuron (the receptor). Only certain neurotransmitters are accepted. If binding is completed, the receptor will let go of the neurotransmitter.

Some specific neurotransmitters are designated to be destroyed by enzymes (complex proteins that affect specific biochemical reactions). Another option is for the proteins to transport neurotransmitters back to the axon from which it originally came. This process, known as reuptake, allows neurotransmitters to be used over again, similar to recycling. The way we might behave, feel, or think is the result of chemical reactions that occur from the receiving or sending of neurons. This nerve pathway sends impulses to reach a destination, such as a gland, a muscle, or an organ.

The synapses alone comprise hundreds of billions of signals transmitting at different levels of intensity. On the neuron's membrane, receptors receive the NT, which reaches the nucleus. The genes are then alerted and the manufacture of new protein begins.

Diversifying the diet in an attempt to load up on amino-acid precursors so that growth hormone can be increased has failed to show any benefit to the brain. Think of all of the advertisements for building up your brain function by pushing diets high in chemicals that form neurotransmitters. They fail due to erratic absorption through the GI tract, and are made up of molecules that do not pass through the blood-brain barrier.

Acetycholine, dopamine, and serotonin are the most important neurotransmitters that bridge and send their messages to more than 100 billion brain cells. Alzheimer's disease is characterized by very low levels of acetylcholine. In Parkinson's disease, a sustained level of dopamine is lacking. Low levels of serotonin negatively impact personality traits and memory.

Acetylcholine (AC)

The brain makes this neurotransmitter from choline and lecithin. Pharmaceutical companies have put out drugs that mimic acetylcholine and drugs that block the breakdown of it. AC-esterase inhibitors allow AC to prolong its activity and to promote and improve memory. These drugs, which inhibit the inhibitor, include Cognex (tacrine), Aricept (donepezil), Exelon (rivastigmine), and Reminyl (galantamine), and studies found them to be effective and safe. Their purpose is to slow down mental decline so that anyone with Alzheimer's or another dementia can remain independent for a longer time. The problem is that the effectiveness is of short duration.

Dopamine

In normal amounts, this neurotransmitter has a stimulating effect on the brain. It is involved in memory, mood, and control of movements, with an emphasis on fine motor coordination. When the level of dopamine falls, Parkinson's disease and its well-known signs of poor coordination and tremor can result. Lower levels of dopamine can also reduce libido.

The neurotransmitter dopamine is broken down by the enzyme monoamine oxidase (MAO). Several drugs attempt to block or slow down the degradation of dopamine by the MAO enzyme. These groups of drugs, known as MAO inhibitors, cause an increase in dopamine levels. Deprenyl (selegiline) is a type-B MAO inhibitor, and its action is directed to the glial cells of the brain. The type-A MAO inhibitor has an overall effect on the body. This type of drug is used in Parkinson's and Alzheimer's disease.

The most popular drug to treat Parkinson's disease is L-dopa (Sinemet), which has been shown to compromise the brain's ability to produce energy and further reduce the production of dopamine. A 1993 research paper related that the chronic use of levodopa (L-dopa) caused an alteration in the cell's mitochondrial respiratory chain. This drug is still sold by prescription. (A nonprescription enhancement for dopamine, described by Dr. Birkmayer, has been previously discussed in Chapter 7.) Dopamine production is enhanced by nicotinamide adenine dinucleotide (NADH), which is sold over the counter. Other studies warn that L-dopa therapy may increase free-radical production and thereby speed up the progression of the illness, causing a worsening of the disease.

Serotonin

This widely studied neurotransmitter is responsible for helping to modulate energy levels, memory, mood, and outlook. Many drugs are designed to enhance serotonin in the brain to help those with lower levels of serotonin who are more vulnerable to aggression, depression, impulsiveness, and even suicide.

Studies in laboratory animals have shown that those with low serotonin levels become more aggressive. Women have been more prone to depression than men; perhaps it is related to a lower production of serotonin in women.

All neurotransmitter and hormone neurons lose the receptors required to activate serotonin with age. Serotonin is necessary for memory and to protect brain cells from excitotoxicity that can destroy neurons. Vitamins B_5 and B_6 are required in the synthesis of serotonin, as well as some fatty acids and other supplements, which can boost serotonin levels.

By enhancing the neuron's fatty membrane, the omega-3s, found naturally in the fish oils of wild salmon and other fatty fish, keep membranes flexible and soft, as opposed to animal fats, which cause rigidity. Rigid fat negatively affects the receptors, and according to Dr. Joseph Hibbeln at the National Institutes of Health (NIH), neurotransmission between receptors cannot be fully effective if the receptors in the membrane are not receptive. Perhaps only 50 percent of a message can get through then, he said.

Studies have revealed that high levels of DHA omega-3 fish oil in the blood are analogous to high serotonin levels in the brain. It is thought the body utilizes this fish oil to manufacture more connections, such as nerve endings and synapses, which in turn elevate serotonin levels.

Serotonin is derived from the amino acid tryptophan. As tryptophan increases in the blood, there is an elevation of serotonin, which induces sleep. People who manifest a depressive disorder, possibly caused by low serotonin levels, also have insomnia.

The serotonin level has an important role in regulating sleep. Prescription drugs such as the selective serotonin reuptake inhibitors (SSRIs) Paxil, Prozac, and Zoloft have a tendency to promote sleep. A more natural way to increase serotonin levels is to supplement with 5-hydroxytryptophan (5-HTP), which connects to serotonin. If you take any antidepressants, however, you cannot take tryptophan or 5-HTP.

REGENERATIVE MEDICINE—BUILDING AN ANTI-AGING PROGRAM

The indicators of aging are not set in stone. Many are reversible and you *can* slow the rate at which you age. Relevant to this chapter, the depletion of hormones is measurable and replaceable. Whether or not to replace them is your choice: If your mind set is to grow old and accept the frailties and cruelty of aging, this information will not be of any use to you. If you wish to age gracefully, however, you have the power to:

- Enhance your mental clarity.

- Enjoy remarkable advances in your general health.

- Improve sexual desire and performance.

- Improve your skin's appearance and texture.

- Increase your energy.

- Keep your immune system at youthful levels.

- Protect your brain cells.

- Restore muscle tone and reduce body fat.

Replenishing is the answer based on a logical and proven program (such regimens are available everywhere—*see* Resources in back). To leap to only one major hormone, such as growth hormone, is not the answer because there are no magic bullets. What works is an *integrated* approach, a coming together of diet, frequent regular exercising, hormone replacement, supplements (antioxidants and others), and overall changes in lifestyle. In combination, all these approaches can renew your functional brainpower and fight aging and degeneration.

Accelerated aging beyond normal, healthy aging is due to the disharmony of neurotransmitters, the depletion of hormones, and an abusive lifestyle. To counter this, I have presented an optimum anti-aging regimen in this chapter and throughout this book. The basis for all replacement plans is to know where you are when you are starting such a progressive program. Your initial step is to find a cutting-edge specialist in restorative medicine. In addition to state-of-the-art blood work and saliva testing (in some cases), testing by this specialist should include:

- Antioxidant panels, full spectrum
- Blood chemistries
- Cortisol levels (saliva testing)
- C-reactive protein
- DHEA
- Estrogens, total
- Ferritin level
- Fibrinogen
- Homocysteine
- IgF-1
- Lipids: cholesterol, HDL, LDL, triglycerides, lipo(a)
- Progesterone
- RBC essential fatty acids
- Testosterone, free and total
- Thyroid antibody testing (if needed)
- Thyroid testing (TSH, free T4, free T3)
- White blood cell functioning assays

After these tests, you might want to follow up with:

- Brainpower supplements tailored to your needs (a multivitamin is insufficient)
- A decision to stop smoking (this is a must)
- HRT (hormonal replacement therapy)
- Positive lifestyle changes

- A nutritional evaluation

- A review of your lab analysis

- Stress management

These are only recommendations. There is no one program that fits all people. It must be customized to your age, gender, weight (body mass index), and existing medical conditions, which are all factored into your goal. Although these guidelines can help you slow your aging process and give you back your youthful energy, only your motivation will get your engine started.

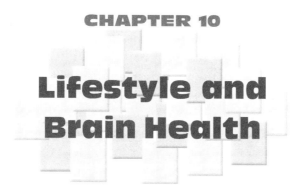

CHAPTER 10

Lifestyle and Brain Health

There are some people that if they don't know,
you can't tell 'em.

—Louis Armstrong

There are compelling reasons to reevaluate your diet; be aware of what surrounds you, and consistently follow a daily regimen. All lifestyle issues impact your brain health and longevity. Now is the time for you to make a strategic plan for your brain empowerment.

BRAIN HEALTH BASED ON LIFESTYLE CHANGES

Seven preventive topics are outlined in this chapter:

1. Avoiding dehydration.

2. Avoiding obesity—a negative condition with serious health ramifications.

3. Avoiding salt—read the labels.

4. Avoiding smoking.

5. Eliminating toxins in your body.

6. Maintaining an exercise regimen to optimize brain health, increase serotonin levels, and benefit you in numerous other ways.

7. Managing stress, anger, and depression in your daily life.

There is a void in the medical community when it comes to seeking out new treatments related to prevention. This is precisely why it is crucial that you take the lead in your own health and brain matters. Most doctors have not addressed the core issue, which is how to strengthen your body and maintain your health to prevent disease. I believe this issue is vital to everyone's brainpower and health, but sadly, too many professionals in the healthcare arena continually overlook preventive ways to achieve these ends when treating their patients. They fail to see the whole health picture of how diet, stress, and lifestyle truly affect their patients.

On the other hand, those of you who maintain a committed and progressive attitude can survive oncoming degenerative illnesses because, ultimately, you are the vanguard of your health. The medical profession cannot take the place of any concerned individual who is serious about his or her daily wellbeing—who knows about the quality of the food being ingested, the quality of the air and water, the working environment, and the amount of stress in her or his life.

1. AVOIDING DEHYDRATION—WATER, WATER EVERYWHERE

Do you drink filtered bottled water all day and night, or are you among the 75 percent of Americans who are chronically dehydrated? Most people in this country consume about 4.6 glasses of drinking water daily, and only 20 percent consume the eight glasses of filtered water that have been recommended until recently. But more than this, people severely dehydrate their bodies by consuming coffee, tea, or alcohol, all of which are diuretics.

Although recent reports have questioned the benefits of consuming eight glasses (64 ounces) of water daily, it is generally considered an essential amount for good health because water (along with oxygen) is the most important nutrient for the human body. All its major systems and critical pathways, including body temperature, waste removal, and joint health, require water for optimal functioning.

Despite the recent reports, it is not news that serious imbalances of fluids and salt occur from drinking too much water or sports drinks (commonly low in sodium) during sports competitions. Following the 2002 Boston Marathon, a twenty-eight-year-old woman died from hyponatremia—excess water diluted her salt level causing her heart to stop. The goal is to replace only the water lost to sweating.

Scientific studies show why consuming adequate amounts of pure water is so important:

1. Joint and back pain occur from dehydration, and eight to ten glasses daily can reduce these ailments.

2. Drinking five glasses of water daily decreases the risk of colon cancer by 45 percent, breast cancer by 79 percent, and bladder cancer by 50 percent.

3. Brain fog (short-term memory loss and poor concentration) can result from mild dehydration.

4. People require the same intake of water in cold or hot weather.

5. The body loses water all day, even while sleeping.

Note: Labels on bottled water may be misleading. For example, a mountain scene with white snow peaks where water gushes fresh from a mountain spring connotes tranquility. If you read the label, however, you'll find the water is actually from a municipal source in Arkansas. The label itself calls the water *purified,* just another word for processed. *Natural* means the water comes from springs or wells with naturally occurring chemicals and trace minerals, which have not been altered during the treatment process. Consumer groups say taste is the primary reason why people purchase bottled water.

The trend toward enhanced water (containing varying degrees of vitamins, minerals, sodium, and sometimes, oxygen) is a case of major marketing skill and overkill. The fact is that oxygen added to water does nothing for the body's cells. As *Consumer Reports* magazine wrote, "The only way the human body effectively absorbs oxygen is by inhalation."

2. AVOIDING OBESITY

The perils of obesity are enormous. This tremendous health risk decreases longevity. The likelihood of multiple other diseases, such as cancer, cardiovascular disease, or strokes, is imminent.

In a speech at an annual meeting of the Endocrine Society, Dr. Stewart G. Albert of the St. Louis University School of Medicine spoke about the low levels of growth hormone that go along with obesity. "When growth hormone is low," he said, "the body tends to accumulate fat, with a loss of muscle, and energy." Fifty-nine obese patients treated with low-dose growth hormone (GH) not only lost weight, but they also increased their HDL (good) cholesterol by 19 percent. Dr. Albert emphasized that growth hormone can supplement, but not replace, the need for diet and exercise.

For many decades I have emphasized the relationship between the lack of exercise and many diseases. Studies have recently shown that moderately intense physical activity can be as effective as a rigid exercise program, which gives hope for those just sitting around waiting for a health catastrophe to occur.

Researchers enrolled 235 men and women in a 1999 study by the Cooper Institute of Dallas, Texas, that was published in *The Journal of the American Medical Association* (*JAMA*). The lifestyle group had 122 participants who learned to fit more physical activities into their daily routines. The other 115 participants used a fitness center for more vigorous exercise. The lifestyle group made changes, such as taking longer walks to office meetings and walking around airports, rather than always sitting and waiting for a plane. The results indicated that physical activity does not require a fitness center or a gym for high-intensity workouts, and that moderately intense activity several times a day for only ten minutes would benefit people (*see also* Chapter 11 on obesity).

3. AVOIDING SALT—READ THE LABELS

Although one teaspoon of salt a day is sufficient, most people consume twice this amount, or even more. Too much salt causes high blood pressure, which is rampant in our culture, and its effects are damaging to the brain, heart, and kidneys. Most of the salt (chemically, a sodium salt) ingested is hidden in packaged goods, and manufacturers are reluctant to change their recipes because that would change the taste. Reducing the salt intake in the average American diet is so important that if everyone were to cut the amount of sodium they presently use in half, hypertension could be reduced 20 percent annually, thereby saving 150,000 lives a year.

4. AVOIDING SMOKING—IT CAN KILL YOUR LIFESTYLE

Smoking is not cool or trendy when the statistics reveal that it killed 5 million people worldwide in the year 2000, mainly from heart and lung diseases. Men accounted for three-quarters of all the deaths, a figure that continues to rise in developing countries, where latest figures show there are 930 million active smokers. Unless effective policies, including intervention, are implemented, the death toll will continue to rise. The World Health Organization (WHO) estimates that tobacco-related deaths will double by 2030.

5. ELIMINATING TOXINS IN YOUR BODY

Toxins are an increasingly common factor in contemporary life so it is important to learn what they are and how to avoid, or at the very least minimize, them.

✗ Cadmium

This mineral, among the most toxic elements, is found in the following sources:

- Art supplies, ceramics

- Evaporated milk

- Fungicides

- Smoke from cigarettes, including secondhand smoke

- Some packaged foods—check labels, especially children's foods

If you need yet another warning about the dangers of smoking, cadmium is the rampant toxin that will force you to quit. Breathing in cadmium (from either your own or another's cigar or cigarette) will compromise your immune system, damage your brain cells, negatively influence your nervous system, and potentially cause lung carcinoma or renal (kidney) failure.

If you insist on smoking, I beseech you not to smoke around your children or others. Adults have the option of leaving the room, but children are captives of your lethal smoke. Although by smoking you are ignoring your life, you should at least be concerned about everyone around you because, without question, secondhand smoke hurts every living being, including your animals.

Everyone has to share the air and it is inhumane to blow poisonous toxins into the air space of others. It has been scientifically proven that multiple poisons damage those in a smoke-filled environment. If this is your lifestyle, you are an agent of deadly delivery.

✗ Mercury

Dental Fillings and Mercury

An overlooked factor that has created havoc with brain health for more than one hundred years is the so-called *silver* in fillings. Your dentists and the American Dental Association (ADA) may not tell you the whole truth about this misnomer for the silver fillings in your mouth (more accurately termed *amalgams* because they are composed of mercury bound to other metals). Although scientific studies have indicated that mercury can be lethal, the reason given for the ongoing use of this toxic mixture for fillings is its ability to adhere to the cavity in your tooth. Consider this daunting statistic, however: The Environmental Protection Agency (EPA) informs us that one single amalgam placed in a ten-acre lake contains enough mercury to contaminate the water and all the fish in it, with predictably harmful results.

There is no such thing as a safe level of mercury. The toxic fillings in your mouth break down into a mercurious vapor that is absorbed almost instantaneously by the brain. If you have silver fillings, any of the following activities will release toxic levels of mercury into your brain:

• Brushing your teeth

• Chewing food or gum

• Drinking hot liquids

• Using plaque removal systems and products

When these actions release mercury into your system, the high fat content of your brain accepts that mercury instantly. And once there, it can interfere with the brain and can create the groundwork for long-term brain dysfunction and disease.

An article I contributed to *Life Extension* magazine in May 2001 indicted mercury in dental fillings as a culprit in diminished brain health. Even moderate levels of mercury in the brain can lead to neurological symptoms, including:

• Cognitive problems

• Headaches

• Imbalance

• Lack of concentration

• Numbness or tingling in the extremities

• Poor memory

It is more than probable that the mercury debacle is seen as suspiciously overblown by the medical establishment because of their own archaic mindset. But their unwillingness to face facts notwithstanding, mercury toxicity from dental fillings can cause other severe health issues, in addition to brain problems, including:

• Abdominal pain

- Anemia

- Endocrine disruption

- Gait disturbance—walking and balance

- Gastrointestinal problems

If you have mercury fillings and experience any of these conditions, I strongly recommend that you ask your healthcare practitioner to test you for mercury levels in your blood, hair, and urine. If the tests confirm that you indeed have mercury toxicity, the following treatments are useful:

- Chelation therapy—this binds mercury to remove it from the body.

- Removing the amalgams (mercury fillings) as quickly as possible.

- Supplementing with DMSA—this element crosses the blood-brain barrier to remove mercury from the brain.

Fish and Mercury

By now, most of you have heard of the health risks posed by mercury levels in most popular fish, including:

- Mackerel

- Shark

- Swordfish

- Tilefish

- Tuna (canned tuna is safer)

The FDA sporadically (and ineffectually) warns consumers of these dangers, but more information needs to be made available. California, for example, has advised grocery retailers to post health warnings about these fish products, but not all stores comply. Most of the problems with mercury arise because power plant emissions containing the toxin wash into rivers and then into the oceans and seas, thereby carrying the mercury directly into the gills of fish that are part of the food supply.

The FDA's ongoing recommendation is that adults eat no more than twelve ounces weekly of the contaminated fish. Children six and under should eat no more than four ounces; children six to twelve years, six ounces; teens thirteen to seventeen years, twelve ounces; and pregnant women should avoid these fish altogether.

A recent warning concerning the additional contamination of fish—including farm-raised salmon—with polychlorinated biphenyls (PCBs) has led to warnings in more than forty states. Mercury and PCBs are known as bio-accumulators—they become more concentrated as the food chain continues upwards and the larger fish consume the smaller fish. The smaller, younger fish are far safer to eat than the larger ones, such as the carnivorous shark or swordfish. Tuna should be limited to two six-ounce cans a week.

Since 1992, researchers led by Susan Schantz of the University of Illinois College of Veterinary Medicine have studied people who have eaten fish in Lake Michigan, generally considered to be a contaminated body of water. Some of their test subjects over age forty-nine have developed problems with learning and remembering new verbal information. This and similar studies suggest that mercury and PCBs may be strongly associated with impaired memory and learning in adults.

Several other scientific papers demonstrate that noxious chemicals are fetal brain disruptors, which lead to neurological abnormalities and learning disabilities, including memory deficits, in children. The following coldwater fish are safer: catfish, cod, flounder, sardines, tilapia, trout, and wild salmon.

Vaccines and Mercury

The effects of mercury in commonly administered vaccines are among the most widespread findings on this toxin. In a recent Associated Press article, medical correspondent Lauren Neergaard wrote that many vaccines contain *thimerosal.* This antibacterial substance containing mercury brings the body's level of this toxic substance up to unacceptable levels in children.

Since children's neurological systems are particularly susceptible to the effects of toxic metals in their body, I strongly recommend that you check with your children's doctor to determine if thimerosal was included in any of the vaccines that were administered to your children. If you find they have excessive levels of mercury, then chelation to remove this toxic substance should be considered.

Toxicity in Other Metals and Minerals

While mercury is a prevailing problem to brain and general health, it represents just one of the many minerals that are toxic to human beings and animals. During your lifetime, you should become aware of the increasing connection between toxic materials and the immune system. Such diseases as chronic fatigue syndrome, fibromyalgia, and multiple sclerosis (MS), plus environmental illnesses and severe allergies, may all be traced to heavy metals that people come in contact with every day. In fact, toxic metal syndrome is now classified as a legitimate disease affecting North Americans.

Neurologists are continually learning more about the effect these metals have on brain development and health. These are the dysfunctions associated with toxic metal contact:

- Alteration of brain chemistry

- Attention-deficit disorder (ADD)

- Cognitive disorders

- Delay in growth

- Poor development of motor skills

Toxins in Household Products

Aluminum

Curiously, some of the most commonly used household products, such as aluminum, are the most toxic to brain health. Aluminum is *everywhere*—in antiperspirants, aspirin, baby powder, baking powder, cigarette filters, commercial teas, cosmetics, dental fillings, table salt, toothpaste, and even white flour. Many pots and pans used in cooking are made of aluminum. This noxious element is also found in canned foods, carbonated beverages, and tinfoil. Perhaps its most pernicious presence is in many infant formulas—it is important to stress how a vulnerable infant's developing body and mind is compromised by this toxin.

Aluminum's presence in the brain has been directly correlated with memory loss, and such diseases as kidney malfunction and osteoporosis are also traceable to high levels of aluminum. Though the problem is widespread, the solution is simple—banish aluminum-based products from your home. Better yet, involve your children in the project, explaining why aluminum needs to be banished. If they understand why aluminum is wrong for their health, they will be on special alert and on their way to becoming responsible for their health as younger people.

Chlorine

A highly effective disinfectant, chlorine has been added to our drinking water for the past ninety years. Most researchers believe chlorine to be carcinogenic because the incidence of carcinoma is higher among people who use chlorinated water than among those who do not.

Although the blood-brain barrier, composed of capillaries, is a protective monitor to keep harmful substances from entering the fetal brain, it cannot fully protect the developing brain in infants and children, which is especially susceptible to chlorine-related neurotoxicity. Pregnant women, too, are especially vulnerable to chlorine consumption (as well as to the chlorine in pool water). Once this neurotoxin enters the bloodstream of the mother and fetus, it continues postnatally for years.

The point I want to emphasize is that public health agencies need to implement strict guidelines about the toxic actions of chlorine. The early developmental brain stages in children need special attention since the toxic burden is much heavier on developing neurons than in the developed, mature adult brain.

Fluoride

The word flouride may impress many people as a miracle substance that has single-handedly prevented cavities for several generations of young Americans. While it is true that fluoride prevents cavities (as does brushing and flossing), its health risks far outweigh the need for it in our water supply.

The deleterious compounds in flouride are the fluorosilicates (silicon and fluoride), which scientists refer to as fluorosilic acid and sodium fluorsilicate. The United States government knows the dangers of fluorosilicates in the water supply, yet it does not acknowledge or publicize them for the public good.

There is startling scientific evidence connecting silica and health concerns, especially those of our brain. *The Journal of Environmental Pathology* clearly states, "Primary brain tumors are among the deadliest of all cancers, with a one-year survival rate of 52 percent. A statistical analysis revealed a significant association between the presence of malignant brain tumors and the concentration of silicon."

Here is more proof. An article in the *Journal of Neurology* relates the association of elevated silicon in cerebrospinal fluid to an Alzheimer's-type dementia—a full 71 percent of people with Alzheimer's showed higher concentrations of silicon in their brains. What happens is, there is a rapid absorption by the brain tissue when fluoride is ingested in water.

Every day you breathe in silica. Not only are silicon and fluoride airborne throughout the home, but you get a double dose when you sleep at night, since your bedding is a transport agent for the silicates. Any matter exposed to the air has silicates, and you inhale them via your carpeting, clothes, and slipcovers. Even if you live in an unfluoridated region, don't think that you and your family aren't exposed to fluorides. You are exposed through air pollution, by eating processed foods, and by using dental products (including most commercial toothpastes).

When fluoride silica is inhaled, these toxicants immediately enter the lungs and bloodstream. From there the path goes directly to the brain, where they do the most damage. The government should be conducting tests to uncover the severe health problem caused by having fluorides in the water supply, but to date governmental agencies have failed to adequately oversee the fluoridation of the nation's water.

The problem gets worse. The American Dental Association (ADA), a group that people generally trust, knowingly endorses toxic fluoride, to the detriment of Americans' health. They are proponents of the use of fluoride in the drinking water and they continue to condone the use of flouride toxins in toothpaste.

The ADA makes millions of dollars every year by endorsing fluoride with their Seal of Approval as though it were the Ten Commandments (probably because it has remained powerful for decades). The ADA states for the record, ". . . for children less than three years old, the maximum suggested amount of fluoride is 0.25 ppm." This is far less than the amount found naturally in the water supply, so for this simple reason, children are allowed to drink toxin-laden fluoridated water. Compound this with fluoridated toothpastes, however, and you can see how it further endangers their development and health.

Of grave concern to everyone should be the fact the ADA continues to receive kickbacks on every cavity filled with mercury amalgams because they own the patent for them. They still advise placing amalgams in the mouth of trusting Americans who are unaware of these toxic materials, even though there are more than adequate substitute materials available today.

Water

The water supply in North America varies dramatically from city to city and state to state. Becoming responsibly informed about the various toxic substances that may be in the water you drink is paramount to securing your family's health. It would be a healthful investment to install filters for the kitchen faucet, the icemaker, and your showerhead.

6. MAINTAINING AN EXERCISE REGIMEN— EXERCISE YOUR BODY, EXERCISE YOUR BRAIN

The media have daily reminders about the many positive benefits of exercise for health and overall well-being. There is ample scientific proof that being physically fit will slow the loss of brain tissue. A recent study of sixty-eight people from fifty-five to seventy-nine at the University of Illinois, Urbana-Champaign, confirms this. These participants ranged from sedentary people to competitive athletes. When their brain activity and composition were measured, the MRIs revealed that the more active test subjects had greater amounts of gray and white matter than the sedentary ones.

In the February 2003 *Journal of Gerontology*, Dr. Stan J. Colcombe, a cognitive neuroscientist at the University of Illinois, states, ". . . just fifteen to twenty minutes of moderate activity, like walking three times a week, is enough to produce a benefit for brain function." And, in fact, there is a mountain of evidence suggesting that physically active people have lower rates of anxiety, depression, and stress than those who are lethargic and sedentary.

The University of Georgia researcher Dr. Rod K. Dishman has shown that exercise increases the concentration of norepinephrine, a hormone that modulates the body's response to stress. Many antidepressant drugs work by increasing the concentration of norepinephrine in the brain.

Mark Southman, Ph.D., at the Indiana University School of Medicine, believes that exercise works to thwart anxiety and depression by enhancing the body's ability to defend itself from stress. He states, ". . . long-term exercise training potentially readjusts the responsiveness of the stress reaction system and makes it more efficient."

In stress, the cardiovascular system communicates with the renal system, which in turn communicates with the muscular system as the circulatory system fills with oxygen. Dr. Southmann explains that ". . . as one becomes de-conditioned, either through sedentary living as forced bed rest due to illness or injury, the physiological stress system becomes less efficient in its ability to respond to a variety of stressors. No other type of clinical intervention forces such dynamic communication as exercise."

This and other research show that even moderate activity, such as walking briskly several times a week, will have a major preventive impact on stress and brain disease. When you exercise, you are exercising your brain too, keeping it primed and functioning optimally for many years to come.

7. MANAGING STRESS, ANGER, AND DEPRESSION IN YOUR DAILY LIFE— DESTRESSING TECHNIQUES FOR BEST BRAIN HEALTH

After many years in my practice, I've seen patients whose complaints of aches, pains, and other symptoms cannot be attributed to a specific disease. It took a long time to recognize the debilitating effects of stress upon the human brain and general state of wellness because the concept, and the word *stress* itself, were not even considered thirty years ago. Up to that time, stress was strictly an engineering term used in relation to buildings and bridges.

I can remember the first time I heard the word stress used in an everyday context, when my middle child, Beth, replied, "I'm all stressed-out, Dad," to my request for her to do some chore in the house. In my mood at the moment, I said unsympathetically, "Beth, here's the definition of stress: When you have a patient on the operating table, his skull open while you explore the deepest crevices of his brain to clip an aneurysm (ruptured blood vessel) and it ruptures, spurting blood profusely in your face—that is stress!" That's how little I understood stress at that time—Beth's stresses were just as real to her as mine were to me because no matter how you interpret stress, it is still overwhelming to you. The stress I feel as a brain surgeon affects my body no more or less than the stress of a cashier at Kmart on Christmas Eve. The burden on the brain is very much the same, no matter what the vocation or position in life.

Stress is not always an acute situation, but it is something that needs to be recognized, prioritized, and adjusted accordingly. Sadly, the type of stress I regularly see in my patients comes from those who say they are just getting by, putting up with an unfair boss, accepting a just-OK marriage, or tolerating chronic pain for years. That many of them have all of these together is worse.

Whatever the source of stress in your life, the overall toll is the same—wear and tear on your body and brain. Stress can exert a positive influence when it compels action, when it forces people to change their lives, their outlook, or their perspective to forge a balance for the better. More often than not, stress acts as a negative influence that is reflected in anger, depression, distrust, or rejection. This is where the mind and body clash, and headaches, hypertension, insomnia, ulcers, and an increased risk of strokes are the results.

How you adapt to the stress in your life makes the difference in your general physical state and brain health. If you fail to deal with your stress constructively, it will manifest in your attitudes and appearance. When stress becomes chronic, small aches turn into major symptoms. People sleep less, smoke more, grind their teeth and develop jaw misalignment and muscle pains, and some binge on alcohol and drugs.

In the ingrained fight-or-flight response, hormones are released when people are highly stressed. These hormones, including adrenaline, cortisone, glucocorticoid, and norepinephrine, are released from the adrenal glands. After entering the bloodstream and the amygdala (an area deep in the brain signaling other parts that something is going on), all this hormonal activity sounds a chemical alarm.

At this point, the glucocorticoid hormones prepare some of the body's internal organs to shut down, while others are alerted to be prepared. Glucose gives the body energy and increases the blood pressure, which then rises to prepare the muscles to deal with this state of emergency. When you're under stress or filled with anxiety, your pupils dilate, the pulse increases, your palms sweat, and your breathing becomes rapid.

If stressful situations occur frequently, you will experience chronic fatigue, exhaustion, and insomnia, which can result from a depletion of the hormone serotonin. If you have chronic stress on a daily basis, the level of hormones will negatively affect your immune system and you will become more vulnerable to illness.

Please note that chronic stress is very different from the kind of sporadic stress you can feel every day. Some people can roll with the punches, whether it's having an accident, marital strife, being a crime victim, or, more traumatically, experiencing divorce, the death of a spouse, the loss of a home or job, or a major illness. Whether the stress times are intermittent or ongoing, from an argument on the phone or from being in shock after a car wreck, it is critical to the brain to manage stress wisely.

It has been discovered that the human immune system is negatively affected by chronic stress. Scientists have documented that caregivers develop severely impaired immune systems and have concluded that stress and depression can permanently alter the immune system.

Adrenal Fatigue and Exhaustion

These two conditions are commonly missed by physicians, and because of this they can be harmful as they can lead to a misdiagnosis, particularly in women. The adrenal glands, located at the top of each kidney, produce many hor-

The Best Strategies to Balance Stress

- Create an environment of goodness. Chinese call this *chi*.

- Do things that give you pleasure. Get involved in something you love. Spending time with things that uplift your passions will rejuvenate your body, spirit, and mind.

- Don't be afraid to say *no*.

- Don't keep bad company. Learn to avoid negative people, situations, movies, and TV. The adage *misery loves company* is true.

- Eat nutritious foods (see Chapter 6).

- Meditate. Studies show that those who meditate and pray enjoy better health—they have less disease than people with no spirituality in their lives. (Studies using an electroencelphalogram (EEG) show an increase in alpha waves, which are associated with quiet receptive mind states, along with lowered stress hormones, lowered heart rate, and lower blood pressure in hypertensive patients.)

- Recharge your spirit with mindful visits around nature, animals, and music.

- Reflect on the good things in your life. Chances are you have much to laugh and smile about. See a happy movie, laugh, dance, or go bowling.

- See a stress-management professional. If you have unknown stress, see a therapist.

- Set realistic goals for yourself.

- Spend time with supportive family and friends. Studies show those who feel emotionally connected to other people and family are healthier in mind and body.

- Try to avoid traumatic news.

mones, plus three neurotransmitters (adrenaline, dopamine, and noradrenalin). The adrenals also produce cortisol, the stress hormone that is released when there is an excess in adrenaline, and that results in anxiety and high stress. A deficiency of adrenaline, on the other hand, results in poor concentration, lack of motivation, low energy, and depression. Continual stress creates a demand on the failing adrenal glands, which adds insomnia to the emotional strife.

The main functions of cortisol are to convert proteins into energy and to counter the effect of inflammation. In the short run, the cortisol effect is positive, but if it remains at high levels for a sustained period of time, it is harmful and destructive.

Chronic elevated cortisol levels can:

- Be destructive to muscle and bone.
- Impair digestion and metabolism.
- Impair mental function.
- Interrupt healthy endocrine function.
- Slow down healing.
- Weaken the immune system.

Conditions related to adrenal dysfunction include:

- Adult acne
- Arthritis
- Chronic fatigue syndrome
- Fibromyalgia
- Hypothyroidism
- Menopause (premature)
- Thinning hair

A Diagnosis

Cortisol levels need to be measured several times a day and at night because there is a diurnal rhythm to cortisol, which requires tracking the day/night pattern. Saliva testing can assess the exact level of cortisol at that moment. It should be elevated in the morning; it should diminish gradually throughout the day to sustain energy, and then drop in the evening to allow restful sleep. With adrenal stress, there will be elevated levels of cortisol during the day and a definite elevation in the evening (the opposite of normal).

Further, adrenal failure causes erratic levels of cortisol, which can be influenced by a diet high in refined carbohydrates and containing too much caffeine. Finally, the adrenals will become exhausted due to the continual low levels of cortisol. If you are emotionally sound, feel balanced, have good energy, and you sleep deeply, you do not have adrenal burnout.

What You Should Do

Your healthcare provider must suspect adrenal dysfunction and request saliva testing. He or she should rule out other diseases or coexisting illness. Nutritional counseling is needed to enrich your diet and reduce stimulants and refined carbohydrates. Supplements, including essential fatty acids, are necessary. Stress reduction and exercise is vital.

Similar to hormone replacement, each individual requires customized low doses of intermittent cortisol, DHEA, and other hormones to see positive results quickly. Reversal of the dysfunction is possible with an accurate diagnosis and your compliance with the regimen.

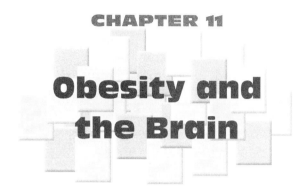

CHAPTER 11

Obesity and the Brain

Every day the fat woman dies a series of small deaths.

—SHELLY BOVEY, BRITISH FEMINIST

No one is born obese, but a confluence of factors in today's society have created the perfect breeding ground for overweight adults, children, and even pampered pets. Big and bigger portions of foods are marketed as the ideal. Oversized fast food is heavily laced with sugar, salt, and fats (hydrogenated oils). Lazy Boy chairs are a perfect fit for lounging around and being vibrated into unconsciousness. Beer commercials deluge devoted television viewers with the subliminal message that it's OK to be slovenly and OK to be nourished primarily by pizza from the delivery man.

Watching TV slows the metabolism down to the point where people expend less energy than if they were doing nothing at all. In a country where everything's "easy like Sunday morning" and billboards everywhere say there are no rules to eating, gluttony is rampant.

Thanks to media bombardment, lethargy has become the rule. For decades, even generations, the American people have succumbed to the convenience-store mentality, and all it has done is encourage a sedentary lifestyle. In the history of the human race, it has never been easier to become immensely fat. As a result, people have gotten fat, so fat that the alarm has been sounded and it is almost impossible to escape the warnings about being overweight. The media put out an endless barrage of misinformation filled with so-called factual warnings on the harmful relationship between obesity and brain health.

Many obese patients have an issue of denial about their health and their weight, and a new study that claims slightly overweight people live a little longer doesn't help. The published results of this study have health professionals alarmed because it does not address the serious health consequences of obesity, and they are afraid that people will use the message as a license to continue being in denial and overeat as much as they please.

Their fears are justified. Reality rules, and the scientifically confirmed reality is that obesity dramatically increases all incidences of the three big primary diseases of the brain, Alzheimer's, Parkinson's, and strokes. Basically a risk factor for all degenerative diseases, obesity is specifically a precursor to cardiovascular disease and diabetes and is linked to brain cancer.

FATVILLE, AMERICA

Let's take a moment to review the facts. The National Institutes of Health states that more than one-half of all American adults are overweight, as defined by the body mass index (BMI), and that obesity is part of the lifestyle of more than 40 million Americans who have a BMI of 30 or greater.

Americans are about eight pounds heavier than they were fifteen years ago. The American Society of Bariatric Physicians (doctors who specialize in the treatment of obesity) estimates that up to 40 percent of women and 24 percent of men are actively trying to lose weight at any one time. Interesting statistic here. There may be just as many overweight men as women, but somehow men do not feel a necessity to lose weight. Even so, Americans spend 30 billion dollars annually on weight-loss products and services.

There is a simple formula to determine obesity. It is: food eaten – exercise = weight gained. Calorie-dense food + sedentary lifestyle = obesity. Common sense says that overeating, sitting for hours, going to bed after eating, and not burning the calories leads to obesity. The calories ingested must be spent by activity. As with any fuel, calories must be burned or they will be stored as fat.

Researchers at many universities are attempting to find out why overweight people eat too much. They know that hunger increases brain activity in the hypothalamus, and they know that following a meal, the hormone insulin signals the brain that the stomach is full, so activity in the hypothalamus decreases. However, in the full stomach of obese people, the signal to the brain is delayed, and they want to know why this occurs.

THE HEALTH RISKS OF OBESITY

• Cancer—breast, colon, endometrium (endometriosis)

- Cardiomyopathy (enlarged heart)

- Coronary artery disease

- Diabetes mellitus, type II

- Fertility problems

- Gallbladder disease

- Hepatomegaly (enlarged fatty liver)

- Hypertension

- Osteoarthritis

- Sleep apnea

- Strokes

DOCTOR, HAVE YOU NOTICED THAT I'M OBESE?

Doctors do not usually discuss the subject of weight because they don't want to offend the person sitting across the desk from them. Also, most of them can't take the time to discuss personal eating habits, and they do not want to treat obesity because it involves behavioral and psychological modification, as well as monitoring the obesity-related medical conditions and the drugs prescribed to treat them. In relation to this, if the healthcare professional you have chosen to help you is obese, you are in the wrong office and should immediately find someone else.

Some physicians are now more aware and can recognize weight-control problems and the lifestyle factors leading to being overweight. Most of them believe, however, that their patients should initiate the topic. As it is, after all, their personal health dilemma, those patients being treated must show an interest in all matters related to their health.

It is essential that your healthcare practitioner show concern and understand your sincere interest in reaching a goal. She or he should help you establish a personal plan. No more excuses; you need to have a specific plan of action. I strongly suggest a food diary as a way to track your diet, lifestyle changes, and weight loss.

Discipline begins with writing down your food intake in this diary every day. This will create awareness of choices, frequency of meals, and size of portions, which will initiate a better lifestyle and lead to weight loss.

GENDER AND OBESITY

The brains of men and women react differently to hunger as well as to satiation. Women have higher rates of eating disorders and obesity than men, and eating disorders contribute to the obesity epidemic. A study reported in the June 2002 *American Journal of Clinical Nutrition* described using the PET scanner to study the brains of twenty-two men and twenty-two women. After the participants endured a thirty-six-hour fast followed by drinking a liquid meal to quench their hunger, they were scanned.

The differences were that hungry men had more activity in the limbic region of the brain, which processes emotion. When sated, women had more activity in the occipital cortex, the seat of vision. Men also had more activity in the prefrontal cortex, which is associated with feelings of satisfaction. From this, it would appear that men derive a more rewarding feeling from eating than women do. Yet there were no gender differences noted in the hypothalamus, the area of the brain responsible for basic physiological responses to hunger and satiation.

"The newly observed brain patterns suggest that men and women differ in how they think and feel about what they eat, rather than in the way they process food compounds," said neuroscientist Yijun Liu of the University of Florida in Gainesville.

CONDITIONS AFFECTED BY OBESITY

Alcoholism

The conditions that characterize alcoholism and obesity are essentially the same. Both of them:

- Affect millions of Americans.

- Are considered lifestyle illnesses.

- Are diseases linked to genetics and a stressful environment.

- Are harmful to health.

- Involve excessive consumption of calories.

- Manifest addictive behavior.

Dr. Todd Thiele, Assistant Professor of Psychiatry at the University of

North Carolina, hypothesizes that part of the brain signals proteins to mediate excessive eating, weight gain, and uncontrolled alcohol consumption. The goal, says Dr. Thielle, is to find intervention strategies. His laboratory explored the role of signaling proteins, the melanocortins (a group of pituitary peptide hormones known to inhibit food intake) in animals. If genetic factors contribute to this behavior, the treatment becomes more complex.

Alzheimer's Disease

Gotenburg University conducted a study of obese women seventy years old and older in July 2003. The body mass index (BMI), a measure of a person's weight in relation to their height, was used to monitor the obesity. The study revealed that obese women over age seventy have a higher risk of developing Alzheimer's disease. Men were not part of the study because too few of them lived long enough to be linked to Alzheimer's. Regardless of gender, however, excess fat is detrimental to the cardiovascular system and damages the blood vessels, thereby reducing the blood flow to the brain, which in turn can trigger Alzheimer's disease.

Brain Hot Spots for Hunger

In another area of research, locating hot spots in the brain might be at the root of the obesity dilemma. An interesting study carried out at the Brookhaven National Laboratory, and published in the July 2, 2002, issue of *NeuroReport,* revealed that the parts of the brain responsible for sensation in the lips, mouth, and tongue are more active in the obese than in normal-weight control subjects.

One of the researchers, Dr. Gene Wang, stated, "This enhanced activity in brain regions involved with sensory processing of food could make obese people more sensitive to the rewarding properties of food and could be one of the reasons they overeat." He and his cohorts found that obese people have fewer brain receptors for dopamine.

In this study of ten very obese volunteers and twenty normal controls, overall brain metabolism did not differ between two groups. To measure the region of brain metabolism, Wang and his colleagues used a PET scanner after injecting both groups with FDG, a radioactive substance similar to glucose that concentrates in the region of the brain where metabolic activity is higher. The PET scanner picked up the radioactive signal to reveal where the FDG radiotracer was located. The computer program produced three-dimensional images that, when highlighted, revealed there was higher metabolic activity in the obese group. These images superimposed onto an MRI of the whole brain revealed hot spots, areas indicating higher metabolic activity in the regions of the parietal cortex where somatosensory input from the lips, mouth, tongue, and taste perception is received.

"The enhanced activation of these parietal regions in obese subjects is consistent with an enhanced sensitivity to food palatability, which is likely to increase the rewarding properties of food. This could account for the powerful appeal and the significance that food has for obese people." Dr. Wang concluded.

These findings suggest that treatments known to decrease palatability could be useful, in conjunction with behavioral modification to reduce food intake in obese people.

Brainpower in Men

A new study suggested that being overweight could increase the risk of mental decline in men. This is the first major study to demonstrate that obesity alone may well decrease brainpower. In a study published in the *International Journal of Obesity*, Merrill Elias, Ph.D., a research professor of epidemiology at Boston University, wrote, "The results indicated that men who are chronically obese have a higher risk of lowered mental ability."

Thinking ability, memory, and learning are all affected by obesity, and the vulnerability in men may relate to the accumulation of midsection fat, as well as to anxiety and depression. Commenting on this, Dr. Charles Belington of the Minnesota Obesity Center said, "Those who value their brainpower should interpret this data as a very strong reason to maintain normal weight."

Cancer

An American Cancer Society study found that overweight and obese people account for 14 percent of all cancer deaths in men and 20 percent in women. Death from most forms of cancer were consistently associated with high body mass index (BMI) and it was concluded that 90,000 cancer deaths could be prevented if men and women could maintain a normal weight.

"Many Americans have not acknowledged the contribution of obesity to chronic disease in general, and to cancer in particular." says Eugenia Calle,

Ph.D., director of analytic epidemiology for the American Cancer Society. She adds that, "Women are very concerned about breast cancer, but few understand that obesity doubles their risk of getting and dying from the disease."

Diabetes

The incidence of diabetes has increased 50 percent in the past ten years. Type II diabetes is the most common form of the disease in middle-aged and older adults, but maintaining a healthier weight via diet and regular exercise can prevent or delay its onset. Research has proven that exercising at least five times a week for thirty minutes provides the health benefit of either preventing or delaying type II diabetes. I certainly encourage management counseling for those who are obese and open to submitting to an appropriate weight-loss program.

Strokes in Women and Men

Physicians have acknowledged that obesity has increased the rate of strokes. Researchers at Harvard used an ongoing study to determine the relationship between excessive weight and strokes. In 1976, The Nurses Health Study had 116,759 women, ages thirty to fifty-five, fill out a questionnaire every two years for twenty years. As reported in 1997 in *The Journal of the American Medical Association (JAMA)*, this study demonstrated conclusively that obesity and weight gain contribute substantially to the incidence of strokes in women. Eating excess portions, hypertension, increased fat in the diet, and smoking all contribute to strokes.

The *Archives of Internal Medicine* published a study in their December 23, 2003, issue that involved 21,414 male participants who were followed up for twelve years and five months. In this study, scientists uncovered a strong link between weight and strokes. Those men who had a body mass index (BMI) of thirty or more were at twice the risk for both hemorrhagic and ischemic strokes, as well as for diabetes and hypertension. A lifestyle of obesity prevention would have considerably reduced their risks for heart disease and strokes.

LIFESTYLE FACTORS AND OBESITY
Breakfast of Champions

Missing breakfast can be a way of saving time in the morning or losing weight, but research equates missing breakfast with an unhealthy lifestyle.

Those who miss breakfast tend to drink more alcohol, exercise less, and smoke more than those who make time for breakfast. The population investigated was also fatter, based on their habit of eating unhealthy snacks for a mid-morning boost.

The children of parents who skip breakfast followed the same route, and research at Helsinki University considered *disordered eating* to be associated with lower education levels, a higher body mass index, and with individuals who take less care with their health. Studies in Britain have shown that schoolchildren who eat breakfast have improved concentration levels.

Diet Sodas and Soft Drinks

The paradox of how a beverage containing no real caloric value could cause weight gain is based on it being loaded with aspartame, which is 180 times sweeter than sugar (*see* Chapter 6). Once it enters the intestinal tract, it converts to aspartate and phenylalanine, both highly excitable to brain cells. This triggers the brain, which signals the taste center to want more sugar. The liver will then store metabolic fuel, such as fat, from the blood. The body, in essence, stops the fat-burning metabolism, making weight gain inevitable. The brain may also send out a signal to replace calories by increasing appetite. This false sweet taste makes the brain cause the liver to store supplies.

All carbonated drinks are dehydrating agents, which lower the oxygen level in the blood. This is not good for the body's performance. In 1950, Coca-Cola was the top dog of sodas, but we only consumed about thirteen ounces a month per person on average. Today people consume fifty-two gallons of this and other carbonated beverages per year, which averages out to every man, woman, and child consuming one gallon of soda every week. The statistics show that 84 percent of all sodas consumed are either Coca-Cola (48.2 percent) or Pepsi (35.9 percent). Then there is the pandemic dumbing down of college students who need *more* oxygenation to their brains, not less. Do not forget the caffeine in soda, another addiction. A study at Pennsylvania State University revealed that many students drink as many as fourteen cans of caffeinated soda a day.

Soft drinks have been effective as grease dissolvers and cleaners due to the phosphoric acid they contain, with a pH of 2.8. This leaches calcium from bones and is a major contributor to osteoporosis. Remember that the slogans, "Coke is it," and "It's the real thing" are indeed true of the negative effects of carbonated drinks on our skeletal structure.

Ice Cream Is FAT!

Many ice creams can contain more fat and calories than hamburgers or pizza. A July 25, 2003, report in *The Guardian* revealed that a single scoop of ice cream can contain two day's worth of saturated fat. Jane Hurley, a nutritionist, found that a Ben and Jerry's waffle cone dipped in chocolate and filled with ice cream had more saturated fat than a pound of spare ribs. She also found that eating a Häagen-Dazs sundae was equal to eating a T-bone steak, Caesar salad, and baked potato with sour cream.

The Center for Science in the Public Interest in Washington, D.C., recommended that calorie counts should be included in menus. The average single scoop of ice cream provides 250–350 calories and a half-day's worth of saturated fat. If you add a cone, fudge, nuts, and whipped cream, that is 1,000 calories and 30 grams of saturated fat—more than in three McDonald's Quarter Pounders!

Sugar and Obesity

Refined sugar is one of the main ingredients of processed foods. It has a long shelf life and does not actually meet the definition of a food, since it does not provide nutrition because it is empty calories—the nutritional value of beets or sugar cane is removed in the processing. Sugar is addictive and can cause mood swings, from hyperactivity to depression. Similar to drugs, there can be withdrawal symptoms.

Sugar added to processed foods negatively affects children even more than adults. Dental decay, immune system dysfunction, infections, and sore throats all occur frequently in children who eat too many sugary processed foods.

American sugar consumption has increased every year because more and more processed foods add sugar. Many breakfast cereals are 50 percent sugar. Colas have up to eleven teaspoons of sugar. Frances Moore Lappé indicts sugar in *Diet for a Small Planet.* She notes that by 1976 the average American was consuming the equivalent of 382 twelve-ounce cans of cola a year, and says, "The next time you reach for a coke, remember that you are about to drink the sugar equivalent to a piece of chocolate cake, including the icing." Tooth decay is rampant. Sugar rots teeth. In his book *Sugar Blues,* William Dufty writes, "Dental researchers have proved that teeth are subject to the same metabolic processes that affect other organs of the body."

Part of the early marketing of sugar supported by the cola companies,

Curtis Candy Company, and General Mills, all members of the Nutrition Foundation, claimed in ads that sugar was a nutrient. In 1973, the National Advertising Review Board found the claim without merit and deleted it in advertisements.

The main target for sugar today is children. An article in the *Los Angeles Times* reported that, in one nine-month period, children were exposed to ". . . more than 5,500 commercials for cereals, candy, and other sugared items." (There was just one ad for vegetables.) Many cereals that are marketed to kids contain large amounts of sugar and deserve to be called candy for breakfast, not cereal.

In *Sugar Blues,* William Dufty explained how the emotions are affected by the intake of sugar. The brain is the most sensitive organ in the body, and the difference between feeling up or down, calm or hyperactive, inspired or depressed, depends in large part upon what kind of food is eaten. When too much sugar is ingested, the glucose balance is no longer in balance. The author uses the term *mortgaged energy* for the aftermath of fatigue and irritability that follows overdoing on sugar.

The latest report from the Centers for Disease Control and Prevention (CDC) says that 61 percent of adult Americans are overweight, and 25 percent are obese with a BMI greater than 30 percent of ideal body weight. Trying to lose weight permanently with a crash diet does not work because most people will resume their former eating habits after the crash. Fasting often depletes the brain of essential nutrients, and starving causes more weight gain when the diet resumes. If glucose is unavailable during a crash diet, the body will obtain a glucose substitute from protein, causing your muscles to dissipate. A carbohydrate diet slows the body's metabolism, which does not return to its former rate when you resume your normal eating habits; therefore you gain weight all over again.

Fat loss comes from burning calories through exercise and weight training, which build muscle. When muscle burns calories, fat loss is increased. You cannot derive sufficient glucose from fat, so if carbohydrates remain unavailable for several days, the body tries to consume protein for glucose instead by producing an alternative fuel source known as ketones (fatty acids). These serve as a glucose substitute to keep the nervous system running, but they build up, causing ketosis—the blood becomes more acidic and therefore chemically imbalanced, causing side effects. The weight loss is dramatic, but it is a loss of water, not fat. In order to obtain a balance for your body, weight loss must be a slow process.

KIDS AND OBESITY

The American Academy of Pediatrics has developed a first-ever policy state-ment regarding childhood obesity. It asks healthcare practitioners to help with obesity prevention and to measure the child's BMI, a height-to-weight ratio. The data so far indicates that 15 percent of youngsters from ages six to nineteen are severely overweight or obese and subject to the looming risks of associated diseases, such as adult-onset (type II) diabetes. A study revealed that breastfeeding may reduce an infant's risk of becoming an overweight child.

Pediatricians are in a unique position to intervene since many of them follow their patients from birth to college. Obesity in young people is a crisis that requires lifestyle modification, for which the child and the parents must all assume responsibility:

- Breakfast—kids who eat breakfast are less likely to be overweight, but skip the sugared cereals.

- Count liquid calories—drinks are loaded with calories and sugars. Push for them to drink water, not juices, which have the same number of calories per ounce as most sodas.

- Eating at home—it's usually healthier, and more likely to include fruits and vegetables.

- Educate the kids about saturated fats and fast food, doughnuts, and snacks.

- Less TV and more exercise—focus on family activities, such as bike riding, swimming, or walking.

- Nutrition begins and ends at home—parents are the models for their children's behavior and children mirror them, so no unhealthy food choices allowed.

- Prudent portions—cleaning the heaping plate down to the last morsel is not the answer.

- School habits—beware of fried foods and vending machines.

- TV time—limit it because exposure to commercials for high-calorie junk food is a negative, and because it is not an active pursuit.

Eating a healthy breakfast allows you to spread calories throughout the day. If it is skipped, doughnuts and sugary pastries are often the substitutes.

In 2004, the Department of Agriculture (USDA) began to issue proper guidelines to schools, but there are still unhealthy meal programs. School lunches have literally been weapons of mass destruction, and are largely responsible for the burgeoning childhood obesity epidemic in the United States. Organizations and parents must be vocal. When I was in school, physical education was not only important, it was mandatory. That is no longer the case, but it should be—the balance of eating and exercise should be reinstated in the school curriculum.

PREDICTING OBESITY

"For humans, the overabundance of food is a very recent problem, just in the past few hundred years," said Dr. Joel Elmquist of Beth Israel Medical Center in Boston. A primary predictor for obesity has been the production of triglycerides, the fat that circulates in the blood. Studies in rats show a huge response after a fat meal—their triglycerides shot up and they were more likely to become obese.

At a meeting of the American Association for the Advancement of Science held at Rockefeller University in New York, Dr. Sarah Leibowitz discussed fat in the diet. She said that if a person's fat intake exceeds 30 percent of the day's total caloric intake, this triggers weight gain because the body is prompted to store the new fat, which makes it crave still more fat to eat, a cycle that could potentially lead to rampant obesity. Dr. Leibowitz is interested in how high-fat food raises the triglycerides, which in turn may activate fat-sensitive genes deep within the brain. The rats with high levels of triglycerides are likely to produce appetite-stimulating substances, and the high triglycerides interfere with the protein leptin that ordinarily dampens appetite.

ASSESSING YOUR RISKS

The National Heart, Lung, and Blood Institute's guidelines and assessment for being overweight include a person's:

- Body mass index (BMI)
- Risk factors for the diseases or conditions associated with obesity
- Waist circumference

BODY MASS INDEX (BMI)

The body mass index (BMI) is a measurement indicating weight status in adults. The BMI is a reliable factor for total body fat. It correlates with body fat, and this relationship differs depending on age and gender. Women with the same BMI as men are more likely to have a higher percentage of body fat. The same is true of older people who may have more body fat than younger adults with the same BMI.

The World Health Organization (WHO) studied the BMI's relationship to your health and the effect that body weight has on diseases and deaths. As the BMI increases, so do the risks for some diseases.

A BMI is generally reliable but there are several limiting factors. One is that there could be an overestimate of body fat, such as in athletes with a muscular build; the other is that body fat could be underestimated, as with older people who have lost muscle mass.

Your waist circumference measurement indicates your abdominal fat. Measure your waist with a measuring tape, holding it snugly around your middle. The risk for ill health increases with a waist of more than forty inches in men and more than thirty-five inches in women. Your BMI combined with your waist measurement assesses your risk for developing obesity-associated diseases.

The BMI Formula

To calculate the BMI:
$$\frac{\text{Weight in pounds } \times\ 703}{\text{Height in inches } \times\ \text{height in inches}}$$

Table 11.1 on pages 218–219 is a simplified way to determine your BMI.

BMI	Weight Status
Below 18.5	Underweight
18.5–24.9	Normal
25.0–29.9	Overweight
30.0 and above	Obese

NATURAL HORMONES AND NEUROTRANSMITTERS TO COUNTER OBESITY

Dopamine and Obesity

The neurotransmitter dopamine is the focus of another promising area of obesity research. An article in *The Lancet*, February 3, 2001, implies that analo-

TABLE 11.1. DETERMINING YOUR BODY MASS INDEX (BMI)

The table below has already done the math for you. To use the table, find the appropriate height in the left-hand column. Move across the row to the given weight. The number at the top of the column is the BMI for that height and weight. Or, use the BMI formula on page 217.

(kg/m^2)	19	20	21	22	23	24
Height (in.)			Weight (lb.)			
58	91	96	100	105	110	115
59	94	99	104	109	114	119
60	97	102	107	112	118	123
61	100	106	111	116	122	127
62	104	109	115	120	126	131
63	107	113	118	124	130	135
64	110	116	122	128	134	140
65	114	120	126	132	138	144
66	118	124	130	136	142	148
67	121	127	134	140	146	153
68	125	131	138	144	151	158
69	128	135	142	149	155	162
70	132	139	146	153	160	167
71	136	143	150	157	165	172
72	140	147	154	162	169	177
73	144	151	159	166	174	182
74	148	155	163	171	179	186
75	152	160	168	176	184	192
76	156	164	172	180	189	197

Body weight in pounds according to height and body mass index.
Adapted with permission from Bray, G.A., Gray, D.S., Obesity, Part 1, Pathogenesis, *West J. Med.* 1988: 149: 429–41.

gous to drug addicts, people may eat more in an attempt to stimulate dopamine pleasure circuits in their brains. And scientists at the Brookhaven National Laboratory have discovered this may be because obese people have less of the neurotransmitter dopamine, which produces the feeling of pleasure and satisfaction. Using positron-emission tomography (PET scanners), it

					BMI below 18.5 is underweight						BMI 18.5–24.9 is normal		
BMI 25.0–29.9 is overweight						BMI 30.0 and above is obese	

25	26	27	28	29	30	35	40
			Weight (lb.)				
119	124	129	134	138	143	167	191
124	128	133	138	143	148	173	198
128	133	138	143	148	153	179	204
132	137	143	148	153	158	185	211
136	142	147	153	158	164	191	218
141	146	152	158	163	169	197	225
145	151	157	163	169	174	204	232
150	156	162	168	174	180	210	240
155	161	167	173	179	186	216	247
159	166	172	178	185	191	223	255
164	171	177	184	190	197	230	262
169	176	182	189	196	203	236	270
174	181	188	195	202	207	243	278
179	186	193	200	208	215	250	286
184	191	199	206	213	221	258	294
189	197	204	212	219	227	265	302
194	202	210	218	225	233	272	311
200	208	216	224	232	240	279	319
205	213	221	230	238	246	287	328

was shown that these obese individuals had fewer receptors for dopamine than people of normal weight. And they also found that, as the BMI (body mass index) increased, the number of dopamine receptors decreased. Further, the study also found that overeating stimulates dopamine in the habit-forming area of the brain, again the same action as in drug addition. One of the

Brookhaven researchers, Dr. Nora Volkow, said, "It is a very basic activation, telling the brain—go for it, take it. Take the food—and it is very powerful."

A dopamine response is significantly triggered by just seeing and smelling favorite foods. The researchers also learned that, in turn, the increase in dopamine triggered hunger and the desire to eat. There still is no perfect pill available because the drugs that regulate dopamine, dexamphetamines, for example, may reduce overeating, but they have also proven to be addictive (just another instance of the harmful side effects of pharmaceutical drugs).

Ritalin, a drug used for children with attention-deficit disorder (ADD), is used in obesity since it regulates dopamine levels, but the studies are incomplete and not yet forthcoming. The only real solution to controlling your weight is to eat more slowly, exercise, reduce the portions of food, be aware of the calories consumed, and practice basic self-discipline.

Ghrelin Signals the Body to Eat

Ghrelin is a hormone that increases hunger by signaling the hypothalamus. Although most of this hormone is produced in the epithelial cells of the stomach—smaller amounts are produced in the kidney, pituitary gland, and placenta—it is delivered to the brain, where it signals the body to eat. Ghrelin receptors are present on cells in the pituitary that secrete growth hormone. Obese people who are dieting and losing weight have increased levels of the hormone in their blood. The more pounds they lose, it seems, the more their bodies demand they eat to make up the difference. Drug companies are looking for a way to reduce the level of ghrelin, thereby reducing appetite.

Surgical removal of the part of the stomach that produces ghrelin has been very successful. In extremely obese people, this radical solution offers one of the most effective means of reducing the urge to eat.

Leptin—Physiological Effects

For a time it appeared that leptin could be the magic bullet to solve the obesity problem. Controlled studies with mice revealed a direct correlation between the lack of leptin and obesity. Research first done at St. Louis University suggests that the protein hormone leptin is secreted from fat cells in the stomach and the placenta and enters the brain through the blood-brain barrier, where it signals the brain that the body has had enough to eat. However, in the obese person, this signal does not get through and the brain does not get the message.

Leptin (from the Greek work *leptor*, meaning thin) is a protein hormone that affects body weight, metabolism, and reproductive function. There are receptor cells in the hypothalamus, which regulates body weight, as well as in T-lymphocytes and the vascular endothelial cells.

Leptin has the specific genetic code of the obese gene, Ob. Studies related to this showed a positive correlation of serum leptin concentrations with the percentage of body fat, and a higher concentration of the Ob gene in fat with obese people compared to thin ones. Adipocytes (fat cells) increase in size by accumulating triglycerides and, therefore, synthesizing more leptin.

The reduced sensitivity to leptin in some people could explain why more leptin is found in obese people. Dr. Jeffrey Friedman, a professor at Rockefeller University, says, "Some obese people may make leptin at a greater rate to compensate for a faulty signaling process or action." He also states, "If resistance to leptin is partial, rather than complete, more leptin may be required for action."

The high rates of regaining weight may be secondary to leptin's signaling ability. "After dieting," Friedman explains, "the levels of leptin drop, suggesting that less leptin is made and available to signal the brain." It is possible that one reason dieters regain weight is that the weight loss decreases leptin levels, which in turn increase appetite and lower the metabolism. Perhaps from these studies, leptin therapy will help people maintain their weight after dieting.

Another problem for the obese individual is the difficulty leptin has crossing the blood-brain barrier, since obesity makes it more difficult. In the lab, fat mice develop a blood-brain barrier defect, but skinny ones do not. To some degree, the defect is reversed with weight loss, but what triggers this process is still unknown, although the neurotransmitter epinephrine is known to stimulate the transportation of leptin into the brains of mice.

There is still another problem with leptin as the cure-all for obesity. Some studies have shown that chronically obese people are leptin-resistant or are immune to the effects of leptin. Theoretically, a leptin drug could avert the problem, but leptin injections are not yet the answer because many people have skin reactions at the site of the injection.

If you have low body fat, your concentration of leptin is low. It enhances the secretion of the gonadotropin-releasing hormone, which stimulates the luteinizing follicle-stimulating hormone from the anterior pituitary gland, and therefore works to regulate reproductive function.

Once leptin is synthesized in the adipose sites, it is secreted and not stored in the cell. The actual trigger to regulate leptin expression is unknown, but it probably is glucocorticoids and insulin.

Peptide YY3-36 (PYY)—Why Obese People Need More

PYY, a shorthand version of the peptide known as YY3-36, is a hormone found in the intestine. It appears to signal satiety, that is, being completely full. Overweight people normally make less of it than thin people. Research continues on why some obese people do not produce enough of it, leaving them without a signal to stop eating.

A research paper in *The New England Journal of Medicine* described the study of twelve obese and twelve lean subjects treated with PYY and saline (salt and water) infusions. Prior to the infusions, the subjects had lower blood levels of PYY. At a buffet lunch two hours after the infusion, the calorie intake of both groups was reduced by 30 percent, and both had a cumulative drop in caloric intake for twenty-four hours. Hormone assays showed that the PYY infusions produced a fall in plasma levels of ghrelin, an appetite-stimulating hormone. However, PYY remains an experimental substance for now and is a doubtful magic bullet since the treatment depends on intravenous injections.

Serotonin—Instant Gratification

Serotonin is a neurotransmitter involved in control of moods, pain sensitivity, regulation of blood pressure, and sleep. Food intake controls the amount of serotonin released. Carbohydrate consumption, acting via insulin secretion and the plasma-tryptophan ratio, increases serotonin release. This does not occur when protein is ingested. The neuron-cell signals are linked to food consumption; it is a feedback mechanism that attempts to keep carbohydrate and protein intake constant.

A popular and appropriate euphemism for carbohydrates is *comfort food.* It accurately describes how the serotonin-carbohydrate connection produces a feeling of gratification. This feel-better gratification is often related to snacks and sweets, such as desserts, French fries, pasta, pastries, potato chips, and all the many foods rich in carbs and fats. The urge for a serotonin-carbohydrate fix can literally be addictive. Nicotine is a good example of this. While it increases the secretion of serotonin, nicotine withdrawal has the opposite effect.

OBESITY DRUGS CURRENTLY UNDER STUDY

Cholecystokinin (CCK)

This is a neuropeptide that is released by the intestine during high fat meals to indicate to the brain that you feel full. Drug companies are researching substances that stimulate the release of CCK as a means of suppressing appetite.

Melanin-Concentrating Hormone (MCH)

This is an appetite stimulant. Injecting the MCH into normal rats increases their rate of food consumption. Several companies are trying to find chemicals that block MCH.

Thermogenesis

This is the production of heat by body cells, which in turn increases the metabolism and burns fat. The chemicals creating thermogenesis are under study regarding their role in the breakdown of fat. They are a potential target for drug therapy.

REDIRECT YOUR LIFESTYLE OR USE MULTIPLE MEDICATIONS— IT'S YOUR CHOICE

A survey regarding whether physicians felt competent to provide counseling for lifestyles came up short, except for smoking. You cannot depend on your doctor to help you change your negative lifestyle of alcohol and excessive eating. Lifestyle changes are determined by you and you alone. Be aware that procrastination is your enemy and motivation will reward you well.

A weight-maintenance program should be a priority after the initial six months of weight loss. Following your successful loss, you can maintain your healthy weight by diet, lifestyle, and physical activity, which should continue on an indefinite basis. If you do use drugs, be aware that their efficiency runs its course, and after one year a drug should be discontinued.

It isn't just people who are putting on excess weight in today's world. The National Research Council in Washington said recently that one-quarter of the pets in this country have the same proportion of obesity as the adults. Junk food is just as harmful to pets as it is to people, and it causes similar risks, such as diabetes, heart disease, and hypertension. The remedies for pets are the same as for adults—fewer calories, smaller portions, and more physical activity.

   To summarize, no drug will ever be a panacea. Losing weight will always involve food choices, portion control, and exercise, and the cornerstone of weight loss will always remain lifestyle changes. By attacking obesity before it gets out of control, you can reduce the need for diet drugs and all their complications.

CHAPTER 12

The Brainpower Plan

I can believe anything, provided it is incredible.

—Oscar Wilde

atients come to me with their shopping bags filled with medications, vitamins, minerals, and out-of-date prescriptions. Before even studying them, I know most of their prescriptions are incompatible with each other and are inconsistent with good medical care.

When someone makes an appointment at the Brain and Memory Institute, we always ask them to bring all the medications they are currently taking or have taken in the last year. Following a complete history, a discussion of nutritional daily intake, a physical exam, a review of previous diagnostic tests, and a thorough look at the contents of the shopping bags, a plan is devised based on the person's *realistic* expectations—realistic because people talk about their ideal lifestyle without necessarily being aware of what is required or how it is going to involve them. For the Brainpower Plan to be successful, self-motivation is required because, for many people, the plan reverses a lifetime of unhealthy habits, and it will take some weeks for their bodies to reverse this damage.

The Institute is about prevention, therefore an analysis of prior health conditions is most important. What if the key complaint is fatigue? Then laboratory work for that complaint is recommended, such as checking the axillary temperatures (under the armpit) each morning for five days (*see* Chapter 9). Blood work and radiological studies may be requested. At times, a thorough nutritional consultation with a certified nutritionist is recommended for a long-term approach to a chronic nutritional problem.

Awareness and up-to-date information is the mission of this book. If you have read it up to this point, you probably have learned a great deal, even developing new brain connections in the process. You can also scratch off some misconceptions regarding aging and cognitive function, as you realize you don't have to deteriorate with these ever-present degenerative conditions. You do not have to end up in a nursing home in the care of a stranger; you can take control of your health now and save your life. Most people do not believe they can affect their own health, but the reality is that everyone is responsible for his or her own healthful longevity. By taking the lead in your health, you can avoid senility and memory loss, and as you feel energized and look better, you will wonder why it took you so long to get it right.

The idea behind the Brainpower Plan is to give you sufficient information to prevent the frailties and infirmities of illness, aging, environmental toxicities, and some lifestyle abuses, which have a decidedly negative effect on your brain. For most people the usual daily diet does not fully enhance the brain, but the genius of the brain is its plasticity, which allows it to change and adapt as a result of environmental influences, vitamins, food nutrients, and varied supplements that nourish it continuously.

DISRUPTION OF NEURONS

Before I discuss the program that helps, I first want to list the factors that cause disruption of neurons. These include:

- A harmful diet
- Consumption of processed food
- Eating out daily
- Excessive calories
- Excessive sugar (glucose)
- Lack of exercise
- Less brain stimulation
- Promotion of free radicals, insufficient antioxidants
- The wrong choices in fat intake
- Toxic artificial additives

THE STEPS TO A HEALTHIER BRAIN

You need to assume responsibility for your brain health. This plan will make a difference in your life and empower you to take positive action to preserve and enhance your brain and its function.

- Avoid processed foods altogether.
- Avoid saturated fats and processed fats and oils. Cold-pressed canola and olive oil are the best. Flaxseed oil is excellent.
- Check your homocysteine blood level. This enzyme is a time-bomb biomarker for heart attacks and strokes. Get a blood test.
- Eat coldwater fish, such as wild salmon. If fish is not for you, supplement with omega-3 fish oil.
- Make your fuel fruits, vegetables, whole grains, and legumes.
- Avoid MSG. Banish this excitotoxin from your diet.
- Avoid Nutrasweet and other aspartame-based sweeteners. They are harmful excitotoxins.
- Reduce intake of refined carbohydrates, such as sugared cereals, white bread, white rice, and white potatoes.
- Water, water everywhere. Drink plenty of water—the body and brain require it. And use bottled or filtered water for everything.

PROTECT BRAIN FUNCTION WITH VITAMINS AND MINERALS

Science has mandated that food alone cannot nourish today's brain. Environmental exposure and overtreated soil with poor absorption and depleted mineral content are just a few reasons why supplementation is so important.

The standard American diet (SAD) is simply not sufficient for optimum health. Your personal vitamin program is about optimizing the intake of supplements to improve your brain and body function. Just as you may have a retirement plan, you need a brain-longevity plan to help you flourish and survive. We are plagued by chaos and stress in this hyper-information, chemically polluted world, which increases the body's nutritional needs.

Minimum recommended dietary allowances (RDA) are not enough for you, and a high-potency vitamin capsule can only contain so much. There are many important additional substances that are not considered established vitamins, such as CoQ_{10}, for example. This is a coenzyme and an important antioxidant responsible for numerous functions in *every* cell, including the production of energy, which is depleted by the anticholesterol statin drugs.

I also recommend L-carnitine, alpha-lipoic acid, and N-acetyl cystine (*see* Chapter 7 for a full discussion of brainpower supplements).

Emotional stress is severely damaging to optimum health. It increases adrenaline, which increases free radicals, causing a depletion of antioxidants that can lead to rapid aging, and ultimately death. And environmental hazards are now recognized as life threatening, as they deplete antioxidants, increase the risk for cancer and the loss of cognition and memory, and cause liver and renal failure and nerve damage.

Then there are prescription drugs, many of which deplete the body's essential nutrients. Even over-the-counter acetaminophen (Tylenol) has unwanted side effects—it depletes glutathione, which is necessary for liver function. Also laxatives, particularly in older people, reduce the absorption of minerals, vitamins, and water.

KEY NUTRIENTS FOR YOUR BRAIN

The following list of vitamins and minerals is a *minimal* guide. If you must take a multivitamin, it should be high potency, with adequate amounts of the following:

Vitamins/Minerals	Suggested Daily Dosage
Vitamin A	5,000 IU
Beta-carotene	15,000 IU
Vitamin B_1 (thiamine)	1.0–1.5 mg
Vitamin B_3 (niacin)	100 mg
Vitamin B_5 (pantothenic acid)	50 mg
Vitamin B_6 (pyridoxine)	75 mg
Vitamin B_{12} (cyanocobalamin)	1 mg
Vitamin C	1,500–2,500 mg
Vitamin E	800 IU
Choline	425 mg
Folic acid	400 mcg
Magnesium	500 mg
Zinc	30 mg

CONCLUDING NOTES CONCERNING NUTRIENTS AND SUPPLEMENTS

If you seriously pay attention to these guidelines, you can expect to experience better brain health in a matter of days or weeks.

- Avoid polyunsaturated vegetable oil, such as corn oil. It has omega-6 fatty acids, which are in excess in the SAD and can cause an inflammatory response in the brain.

- Be sure to take in essential antioxidants, including alpha-lipoic acid, bioflavonoids, CoQ_{10}, and ginkgo biloba.

- Eat fruits and vegetables. Fruits contain antioxidants—berries, cherries, dried raisins, and prunes particularly. Vegetables, such as broccoli and spinach, also contain antioxidants.

- Consult a nutritionally aware health professional to check your vitamin B_{12} level.

- Consider natural bio-identical hormone replacement—estrogen, progesterone, testosterone, and thyroid, which reverses and strengthens many systems in the body and brain.

- No more slurpies—just say *tea*. Black tea has the most antioxidants; herbal teas are not high in antioxidants.

- Take 300 mg of phosphatidylserine a day.

- Get active. Physical exercise improves cerebral blood flow for brain function.

- Get a good night's rest. Sleep is vital. Sleep disruptors include alcohol, all caffeinated drinks, and eating dinner late.

- Concentrate on smart fats, including omega-3 fatty acids (DHA) fish oil capsules and flaxseed oil.

- Reduce sugar consumption. Sugar is extreme in the SAD, and creates cellular brain damage and insulin resistance. Excess sugar defeats brain function and its ability to promote cognition.

- Avoid foods that contain trans-fatty acids, including doughnuts, fast foods, fries, and margarine. They are horrific to brain circulation.

Future Visions— Starting Now

Hypotheses and trends come and go, that is how science works. Biochemistry and nutrition are now front and center in the prevention of degenerative diseases. Every system of the body is intertwined and involved in complex relationships with each other.

The noted nutritional biochemist, Jeffrey S. Bland, Ph.D., described a *metabolic biotransformation* involving the reactions of neurotransmitters and hormones, and genetic expression, as being responsible for regulating your physiological health. In this book, I discuss many processes and risk factors over which you alone have control. In the present environment, nutritional factors and genes have the power to influence the promotion of longevity and brain health, but ultimately it is up to you to take back your life.

Science continues to move forward and does not remain in the moment. It is the continuum of progressive data learned from the past that looks forward to the future.

In the past decade, this country has had an obesity explosion that continues to balloon, and hunger is now being studied at the molecular level. I believe in the near future there will be a kind of safe pill for those who abuse themselves by overeating. A study published in *The New England Journal of Medicine* in August 2003 stated that a protein found naturally in the body may indeed put scientists a step closer to developing a natural and effective diet pill.

There will be preventive medicine based on your own DNA. Diseases may occur, but the medicine will be customized to fit your specific need.

Cell therapy, genetically engineered, will be able to replace or repair diseased organs. Stem cells will be used to cure degenerative disease and intractable cancer.

The recently discovered specific genes for aging may be modulated, so the

231

aging process can be truly slowed. Retirement might not be in people's future when living to 150 years is a reality. Think of the possibilities.

The human genome may always have faults or defects, but these will be reparable. And what about human intelligence? Maybe you will be able to purchase a gene program. Biological intelligence may not be fixed when information processing continues to grow exponentially with computational technology.

If the scientific community works with individual genotypes, even mental illness could be fully treatable. But genetic information has to be used for the good only. The social, economic, and moral issues it raises will not be easy to legislate, but I believe science will prevail.

Brain-specific replacement of damaged or dead neurons may be dependent on drugs being investigated at this time, which may turn out to stimulate the brain to enhance and replace its own cells. Neurogenesis (the birth of new neurons) is controlled by growth factors, some of which are naturally occurring, and have the ability to stimulate new neurons or glial cells (cells that support the neurons).

Additional growth factors are under competitive and intense investigation. The hope is that one day these growth factors may be administered as a useful drug to treat brain disorders or replace the injured portions of the brain and spinal cord.

Emerging therapies for optimal brain function will help restore, renew, and regenerate—enriching your mind, memory, and mood.

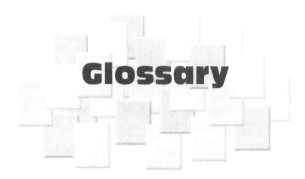

Glossary

Acetylcholine. A neurotransmitter involved in memory and learning; low levels of acetylcholine in the brain are typical in those with Alzheimer's disease.

Acetyl-L-carnitine (ALC). A nutritional supplement derived from the amino acid L-carnitine. ALC protects neurons (nerve cells) by boosting the production of nerve growth factor, enhancing the activity of acetylcholine, neutralizing free radicals, and stabilizing cellular membranes.

Adaptogen. A substance that safely increases resistance to stress and balances body functions. Ginseng is an example of an adaptogen.

Adrenal gland. One of two organs situated above the kidneys and comprised of a medulla and cortex. The adrenal medulla produces the hormones epinephrine and norepinephrine, which play a part in controlling heart rate and blood pressure. The adrenal cortex produces steroid hormones that have numerous functions throughout the body.

Adrenaline. *See* Epinephrine.

Advanced glycation end products (AGEs). Chemically altered proteins formed as a reaction to excess sugar. AGEs can cause damage to the endocrine, immune, and nervous systems. *See also* Glycation.

Aerobic exercise. Includes cycling, jogging, and swimming, activities during which the oxygen rate reaching the muscles keeps pace with the rate it is used up.

Age-associated memory impairment. A progressive decline in memory and cognitive function, generally beginning between the ages of forty and fifty. This type of memory loss is not to be confused with Alzheimer's disease or other forms of dementia.

Allicin. A pungent, sulfur-containing compound that becomes beneficial when garlic is minced, crushed, swallowed, and digested. It has been shown to lower blood pressure, cholesterol, and the risk of cancer.

Alpha waves. Slow, low-amplitude brain waves that indicate a calm, relaxed state of wakefulness.

Alpha-linolenic acid. An essential fatty acid of the omega-3 family that converts to docosahexaenoic acid (DHA) and eicosapentaenoic acid (EPA), which are important for proper brain function.

Aluminum. A light metallic element harmful to the body that enters the body through ingestion or absorption of antacids, antiperspirants, cooking utensils, and food additives, such as potassium alum, which is used to whiten flour.

Alzheimer's disease (AD). A progressive type of dementia, characterized by confusion, disorientation, and deterioration of behavior, memory, language skills, and personality. It is not to be confused with age-associated memory impairment.

Amino acids. The building blocks of proteins. The value of protein is that it is broken down into its amino acids by hydrochloric acid in the stomach and then by digestive enzymes in the small intestine. There are twenty amino acids that make up the protein in humans—twelve are made by the body (nonessential) and eight must be obtained by diet (essential).

Amygdala. The region of the limbic system that adds emotional color to experiences and memories.

Anaerobic exercise. A brief, high-intensity workout, such as sprinting, that relies on a series of biochemical reactions to obtain energy from the stores of sugar and fat in muscle.

Andropause. The gradual decline in testosterone levels that causes loss of muscle mass, as well as reduced energy, libido, and motivation in men around the age of forty-five or fifty. It is similar to the female menopause.

Aneurysm. The ballooning of an artery due to the pressure of blood flowing through a weak area. An aneurysm can occur anywhere in the body, but most often occurs in the brain and aorta.

Antioxidant. A substance, such as vitamins A, C, E, or the mineral selenium, that helps protect cells by neutralizing toxic free radicals.

APOE4. A variant form of a gene used to make the protein apolipoprotein E. It occurs more often in people with Alzheimer's disease than in the general population.

Apolipoprotein E. A lipoprotein (fat and protein compound) that carries cholesterol in the blood and appears to play some role in the brain.

Arachidonic acid (AA). An omega-6 essential fatty acid that is a structural component of brain cells. When not balanced by other fatty acids, AA can form highly inflammatory and sometimes damaging prostaglandins.

Arginine and ornithine. Two amino acids, usually prepared and sold in combination. Arginine is the building block needed by the anterior pituitary gland in the production of human growth hormone. Ornithine serves as a reserve supply because it is easily converted to arginine.

Ascorbic acid (vitamin C). This potent water-soluble antioxidant helps prevent diseases caused by cellular damage from free radicals, for example, cancer, cataracts, and heart disease. Among its many benefits, it is an important factor in strengthening and maintaining the immune system.

Aspartame (NutraSweet). An artificial sweetener derived from the amino acids aspartate and phenylalanine. This excitotoxin is a commonly used food additive that overstimulates brain neurons and has been implicated in dizziness, headaches, mood changes, seizures, and vision problems.

Atherosclerosis. This is a narrowing of the arteries and subsequent reduction in blood supply due to fatty deposits that thicken the inner layers of the artery walls.

Axon. The nerve fiber of a neuron that transmits impulses to the dendrites of another neuron.

Beta amyloid. This protein is found in dense deposits in the senile plaques and neurofibrillary tangles that are characteristic of Alzheimer's disease.

Beta-carotene. The precursor to vitamin A. It is an antioxidant that helps neutralize free radicals. It may help prevent atherosclerosis and cervical cancer. It is an immune-system booster and appears to protect against respiratory diseases and environmental pollutants.

Beta waves. These are irregular brain waves that are higher in frequency than alpha waves; they occur when a person is awake and mentally alert.

Blood-brain barrier (BBB). This is a dual layer of brain capillaries that prevents certain disease-causing organisms, drugs, and toxins from making their way to the central nervous system via the bloodstream. It blocks all but the smallest molecules from entering the brain. The molecules of some drugs are too large to pass through the barrier.

Borage oil. This contains a linoleic acid that reduces the risk of atherosclerotic heart disease.

Boron. A trace mineral that aids in the synthesis of steroids, particularly the estrogens and testosterone. It may help prevent osteoporosis and memory loss.

Broca's area. The region in the frontal cortex of the brain involved in the production of speech.

Calcitonin. A hormone that slows the rate at which bone is broken down, thus decreasing the amount of calcium that is leached from the bone and dissolved in the blood.

Calcium. The most plentiful mineral in the body. Mainly found in the bones and teeth where it helps maintain their strength. Vitamin D is required for the absorption of calcium. Calcium with magnesium keeps the electrical heart rhythm pulsing regularly.

Carboyhdrates. A group of organic compounds, including sugars, starches, gums, and celluloses. They are a major energy source in the diet. There are complex and simple forms. Complex carbohydrates are obtained from grains and other whole foods comprised of hundreds or thousands of sugar units linked together in a single molecule. Candy is a simple carbohydrate with sugars linked to one molecule.

Cell body. The central portion of a nerve cell that contains the nucleus and is responsible for making proteins and membranes.

Cerebellum. A region of the brain that lies at the back of the head just behind the brain stem. It regulates coordination, equilibrium, movement, and muscle tone.

Cerebral cortex. The area of the brain that is most involved in language, learning, and reasoning. Also called the neocortex, it is a thin layer that covers the cerebrum.

Cerebral infarct. A loss of oxygen to the brain that can promote strokes.

Cerebral vascular insufficiency. Inadequate blood flow to the brain.

Cerebrovascular accident. *See* Strokes.

Cerebrum. The largest and uppermost portion of the brain, consisting of a right and left hemisphere. Also known as the mammalian brain, it is crucially involved in emotion, memory, and thought.

Cholesterol. A substance produced by the body or derived from food that is a precursor to steroid hormones. Cholesterol is a crucial component of cell membranes and the myelin sheaths that protect and insulate the axons of nerve cells. High levels are associated with an increased risk of heart attacks and strokes.

Choline. An essential nutrient in the manufacture of the neurotransmitter acetylcholine that plays a crucial role in memory for some people who have mild to moderate dementia or Alzheimer's disease; also required for healthy cell membranes and aids in the production of HDL (good) cholesterol.

Cholinesterase. An enzyme found primarily at nerve endings. It catalyzes (breaks down) various cholines, including acetylcholine, a neurotransmitter, into acetic acid and choline. It occurs mostly in blood plasma, the liver, and the pancreas.

Chromium picolinate. A trace mineral that is deficient in most diets. It can lead to sugar intolerance (diabetes). When the amount is sufficient, it helps to increase muscle mass and prevent diabetes and heart disease. It is necessary for the breakdown of sugar and the metabolism of fat.

Chromosomes. Threadlike structures in the nucleus of cells that contain the genetic information that directs the growth and functions of the body.

Circadian rhythm. A pattern of activity, such as sleep/wakefulness, that is based on a twenty-four hour cycle.

Citicoline. A naturally occurring nootropic that helps boost the production of acetylcholine and phosphatidylcholine. It also enhances electrical activity in the brain, protects brain cells from damage caused by insufficient blood or oxygen, and may improve memory and learning.

Coenzyme. The active or working form of a vitamin essential to metabolism.

Coenzyme Q_{10} (CoQ_{10}). An essential nutrient for energy production in the mitochondria of all cells in the body, including brain cells. It is also a potent antioxidant.

Corpus callosum. The band of nerve fibers that connects the right and left cerebral hemispheres.

Corticosteroid. A hormone secreted by the adrenal cortex that influences key processes in the body, including metabolism and blood pressure. Chronic stress can result in high levels of corticosteroids that impair immunity and accelerate aging of the brain.

Cortisol. A type of cortocosteroid. When chronically elevated, it can cause injury and death to brain cells. The levels are elevated in the fight-or-flight response.

Cytokine. Any of several regulatory proteins, such as interleukins, released by cells of the immune system. They act as intercellular mediators in the generation of an immune response.

Degenerative disease. The chemical change in deteriorating cells and tissues which makes them less functional.

Dehydroepiandrosterone (DHEA). A steroid hormone from which estrogen and progesterone can be derived. DHEA enhances immune functions and helps counteract the detrimental effects of stress on brain cells. Low levels are associated with Alzheimer's disease, cancer, cardiovascular disease, diabetes, and obesity.

Delta waves. The slowest type of brain waves, indicating a state of deep, dreamless sleep.

Dementia. A progressive mental disorder characterized by confusion, disorientation, impaired cognition and memory, and personality disintegration. Dementia may be reversible or irreversible, as in the case of Alzheimer's disease.

Dendrites. Branch-like extensions of a neuron that receive messages from axons.

Deprenyl. A drug that prevents the destruction of the neurotransmitter dopamine. It is used to treat Alzheimer's disease, depression, loss of libido, and Parkinson's disease.

DHA. *See* Docosahexaenoic acid.

DHEA. *See* Dehydroepiandrosterone.

Dimethylaminoethanol (DMAE). The principal fatty acid of the brain. It is involved in memory and nerve-cell communication and is manufactured from dietary or supplemental omega-3 fatty acids. DHA deficiencies are associated with an increased risk of Alzheimer's disease, dementia, and memory loss.

Docosahexaenoic acid (DHA). The primary structural component of brain tissue. It is crucial for neurotransmitter function. It is an omega-3 fatty acid found in egss and cold-water fish, such as salmon, sardines, mackerel, and tuna.

Dopamine. Energizing neurotransmitter that affects memory, mood, motor control, and sex drive.

Eicosapentaenoic acid (EPA). A fatty acid that enhances brain function by improving blood flow and delivery of oxygen and nutrients to the brain. EPA is manufactured in the body from dietary or supplemental omega-3 fatty acids.

Electroencephalograph. An instrument for recording brain-wave activity.

Endorphins. Neurotransmitters produced by the brain in response to stress. They elevate mood and reduce the perception of pain.

EPA. *See* Eicosapentaenoic acid.

Epinephrine. The chief hormone produced by the adrenal gland. It regulates heart rate and metabolism, and helps initiate the fight-or-flight response during periods of stress.

Essential fatty acid (EFA). A type of polyunsaturated fatty acid required for proper growth, maintenance, and functions of the body. EFAs are essential to the manufacture of cell membranes, myelin sheaths, and prostaglandins. They can only be obtained from the diet. *See also* Omega-3 fatty acid, Omega-6 fatty acid.

Estradiol. The most potent naturally occurring form of human estrogen.

Estriol. A relatively weak naturally occurring form of human estrogen.

Estrogen. A steroid hormone that promotes the development of female secondary sex characteristics and also plays and important role in bone health, brain function, and cardiovascular health.

Exhaustion. Final stage of the stress response in which stress hormones are depleted and organ systems begin to fail.

Fight-or-flight response. The body's reaction to a dangerous or threatening situation where it prepares to either stay and fight the danger or run from it.

5-hydroxytryptophan (5-HTP). A precursor to the neurotransmitter serotonin that is used therapeutically as an antidepressant and sleep aid. It is synthesized in the body from tryptophan, or derived from the seeds of the West-African plant *Griffonia simplicifolia.*

Free radicals. Highly reactive molecules that bind to, and destroy, cellular compounds, including cell membranes, DNA, and proteins.

Frontal lobe. The portion of the cerebrum that significantly influences personality and is involved in higher mental activities, including abstract reasoning, judgment, and planning.

Gamma-aminobutyric acid (GABA). A calming neurotransmitter that prevents the brain from being overwhelmed by excessive stimulation.

Gamma-linolenic acid (GLA). The omega-6 fatty acid that produces protective anti-inflammatory prostaglandins.

Gene modulation. A transition of gene expression.

Ginkgo biloba. An herb with powerful antioxidant properties that can help improve blood circulation and delivery of oxygen and nutrients to the brain.

Ginseng. A class of herbs that balance bodily functions and increase physical and mental energy and stamina. Popular types include American ginseng (*Panax quinquefolius*), *Panax ginseng,* and Siberian ginseng (Chinese).

Glial cells. Brain cells that provide antioxidant properties, which can help improve blood circulation and delivery of oxygen and nutrients to the brain.

Glucagon. A hormone manufactured by the pancreas that plays a vital part in monitoring sugar levels in the blood.

Glucocorticoid. An adrenal hormone, such as cortisol. Excessive levels, commonly produced under chronic stress, may be toxic to the brain.

Glutamate. An amino acid that acts as an excitatory neurotransmitter in the brain. When balanced with GABA, glutamate helps keep the brain in balance.

Glutamine. The precursor of glutamic acid, which serves the brain by neutralizing excess ammonia, thus creating a clearer space for brain activity. Glutamine may improve IQ, and alleviate fatigue, depression, and impotence, as well as promote healing.

Glutathione peroxidase. An enzyme with an important role in protecting against free-radical damage.

Glycation. The reaction between cellular proteins and excess glucose that results in chemically damaged proteins. It is considered one of the four leading causes of aging.

Glycemic index. A list of values assigned to foods to denote the rate at which blood-sugar levels rise after they are eaten. A high-glycemic-index value indicates a food that produces a *rapid* rise in blood sugar, followed by a dramatic fall. A low-glycemic-index value indicates a food that produces a *gradual* rise and fall in blood sugar.

Hippocampus. The region of the limbic system that plays a role in converting new information into long-term memories.

Homocysteine. A byproduct of normal amino-acid metabolism. High levels can become toxic and can accelerate Alzheimer's disease, atherosclerosis, cancer, and other degenerative conditions, as well as impair circulation and stimulate free-radical damage to cells.

Hormones. Hormones serve as molecular messengers that are governed by the brain and regulate all the glands.

Human growth hormone (hGH). The hormone responsible for maintaining the tissues of the body in a state of vitality. It diminishes as you grow older, until age sixty, when it is usually absent. Many of the aches and pains of aging are a result of diminishing levels of this hormone.

Huperzine A. An extract from club moss (*Huperzia serrata*) that inhibits the breakdown of the neurotransmitter acetylcholine. It has been demonstrated to enhance concentration and memory.

Hydergine. A nootropic widely prescribed in Europe that enhances blood and oxygen supply to the brain, protects against free-radical damage, speeds up brain metabolism, and may enhance the effects of nerve-growth factor and promote the growth of dendrites.

Hypertension. A condition in which blood pressure consistently increases. Hypertension often has no symptoms in its earliest stages, but may eventually cause congestive heart failure, a heart attack, or a stroke.

Hypothalamus. The part of the brain's limbic system that regulates blood pressure, body temperature, heart contractions, hunger, respiration, sleep/wake cycles, and thirst. It also controls the endocrine system's functioning and is the center for emotional response and behavior.

Hypothyroidism. A condition caused by deficient activity of the thyroid gland. Symptoms include general loss of vigor, lethargy, lowered metabolic rate, and weight gain.

Hypoxia. Inadequate supply of oxygen to an organ or body part.

Inflammation. Acute inflammation is a short-lived response by the immune system to tissue injury or invasion by bacteria or other harmful agents that serves to protect the site and promote healing. Chronic inflammation is linked to numerous diseases of aging, including Alzheimer's disease, arthritis, cardiovascular disease, dementia, and strokes.

Insulin. A hormone secreted by the pancreas to lower blood-sugar levels.

Insulin resistance. A metabolic disorder where the body produces adequate insulin but is unable to utilize it correctly to maintain healthy blood-sugar levels.

Interleukins. A type of cytokine which mediates an immune response by interacting with a specific cell-surface receptor responsible for regulating immune and inflammatory responses.

Iron. A metal that is essential for the formation of red blood cells and the metabolism of vitamin E. In excess, iron may be a strong catalyst in free-radical production and may aid in depositing plaque in blood vessels.

Ischemia. A decreased supply of oxygenated blood to an organ or body part.

Isoflavones. Plant estrogens that are chemically structured like estrogen and have similar effects, but are weaker. Two primary isoflavones are in soybeans.

Kava. An herb (*Piper methysticum*) that targets the limbic system to help relieve anxiety and produce a sense of calm and peacefulness without impairing concentration or memory.

L-arginine. A nonessential amino acid that can stimulate the release of growth hormone. It may be an effective immune enhancer and may help in the nutritional treatment of male infertility.

L-carnitine. An amino acid that transports fatty acids across the mitochondrial membrane to be utilized as sources of energy.

Lecithin. A naturally occurring compound that is rich in phosphatidylcholine, an important component of nerve-cell membranes.

Left hemisphere. Left side of the cerebrum. This hemisphere controls the right side of the body and is the dominant region for language, logic, and mathematical abilities in the majority of people.

L-glutamine. An amino acid that helps control alcohol craving, counteracts depression, energizes the mind, and inhibits senility.

Limbic system. An area deep in the brain consisting of the amygdala, hippocampus, hypothalamus, pituitary gland, and thalamus. It mediates emotional responses and is involved in memory processing.

Linoleic acid (LA). An essential fatty acid that can help prevent hardening of the arteries, heart disease, high blood pressure, and multiple sclerosis. It also aids in lowering cholesterol levels, has a positive effect on sex-hormone response, and is important for healthy skin.

Long-term memory. The durable memory of personal events, knowledge of the world, and procedural knowledge.

Luteinizing hormone. This hormone stimulates ovulation and prepares a woman's body for pregnancy. In men, it triggers the testes to produce male sex hormones.

Lysine. An essential amino acid found in food protein that is needed for enzyme production, normal growth, and tissue repair. It aids in the metabolism of fat, alleviates some infertility problems, has antiviral properties, helps to stimulate the immune system, and inhibits the herpes virus.

Magnesium. A mineral involved in the metabolism of carbohydrates and protein. It acts as an antagonist to calcium and tends to prevent calcium stones in the kidneys and gallbladder, as well as the calcium deposits of arteriosclerosis. Magnesium is also required for the proper functioning of the central nervous system. Alcohol depletes magnesium and this is a problem in alcoholism that can lead to seizures.

Manganese. A mineral involved in diverse enzyme systems. It is important to the proper use of biotin, thiamine, and vitamin C, and the normal functioning of the central nervous system, proper digestion, the production of thyroxin, and sexual function.

Medulla. The portion of the brain stem that contains the brain's cardiovascular and respiratory centers.

Melatonin. A hormone secreted by the pineal gland in response to changes in temperature and light that plays a key role in regulating sleep.

Menopause. A gradual decline in levels of estrogen and progesterone that causes the cessation of menstruation. Lowered levels of these hormones have an adverse effect on bone density, cardiovascular health, and cognitive function.

Metabolism. This is the rate at which the body uses energy.

Methionine. A sulfur-containing amino acid that protects against cardiovascular disease.

Methyl donor. A nutrient, such as vitamin B_{12}, that contributes a methyl group (CH-3) derived from methane.

Methylation. The body's primary mechanism for neutralizing harmful compounds by combining them with methyl groups. This bioactivity or reaction is associated with degenerative diseases, including Alzheimer's disease, cancer, and heart disease.

Microglia. Supporting cells of the central nervous system that help protect the brain from neural damage and inflammation.

Mitochondria. Components in the cell's cytoplasm that generate energy. Contains DNA and RNA.

Monoamine oxidase (MAO) inhibitor. A drug, such as deprenyl, which raises levels of dopamine by blocking the activity of an enzyme that breaks down this neurotransmitter.

Monosodium glutamate (MSG). A food additive that increases levels of glutamate, an amino acid that acts as an excitatory neurotransmitter in the brain. It is considered a neurotoxin due to its harmful effects on nerve cells.

Monounsaturated fat. A type of fat found in vegetable oils, such as canola, olive, and peanut. It is liquid at room temperature and relatively stable when exposed to heat. The body can produce this type of fat.

Motor cortex. The portion of the cerebrum that conveys signals for action from the brain to the body.

MSG. *See* Monosodium glutamate.

Myelin sheath. The fatty covering of most nerve fibers that protects and insulates them. It increases the transmission speed of nerve impulses.

Nerve growth factor (NGF). A hormonelike protein that promotes the growth and maintenance of neurons.

Neuroglia. *See* Glial cells.

Neuron. The basic nerve cell of the nervous system, composed of a cell body, one or more receptive extensions (dendrites), and a transmitting extension (axon).

Neurotoxins. Poisonous substances, such as food additives, heavy metals, and some drugs, that can negatively affect the brain and nervous system.

Neurotransmitter. A chemical substance released from the end of a neuron during the propagation of a nerve impulse that relays information from one neuron to another. Serves as the basis of communication between nerve cells.

Niacin (vitamin B$_3$). A potent vasodilator. It enhances energy production and the normal functioning of the nervous system, helps lower cholesterol, may boost the effects of chromium, promotes healthy skin, and protects against sun damage. It helps maintain a balanced neurochemistry, promotes healthy colon function, and provides protection against the development of arteriosclerosis.

NMDA (N-methyl-D-aspartate). A type of excitatory amino-acid receptor.

Nootropics. A class of drugs that enhances cognition, concentration, memory, and perception.

Norepinephrine. A neurotransmitter and adrenal hormone that helps lay down new memories and transfer memories from short-term to long-term storage in the brain. It also changes blood flow patterns and raises blood pressure during periods of acute stress.

NutraSweet. *See* Aspartame.

Occipital lobe. The portion of the cerebrum that governs vision.

Omega-3 fatty acid. A type of polyunsaturated fatty acid found in fish oil and flaxseed oil. ALA, DHA, and EPA are omega-3 fatty acids.

Omega-6 fatty acid. A type of polyunsaturated fatty acid found in proteins and most seed oils. GLA is an omega-6 fatty acid.

Oxidation. The generation of highly reactive molecules called free radicals as a consequence of normal cellular processes. These molecules damage cell membranes, DNA, and proteins, and they accelerate the aging process.

Pancreas. One of the glands of the endocrine system. It controls blood sugar (glucose) by producing insulin, which decreases glucose levels, and glucagon, which increases them. Digestive enzymes are also produced in the pancreas.

Parietal lobe. The portion of the cerebrum that helps process information received from the senses.

Parkinson's disease (PD). A degenerative neurological disorder caused by a decrease in brain levels of the neurotransmitter dopamine. It is characterized by muscle tremors, a shuffling gait, and weakness.

Peptide. A compound of two or more amino acids.

Perimenopause. A period of about five years before the onset of menopause when some menopausal symptoms, such as hot flashes and irregular bleeding, occur sporadically.

Phenylalanine. An amino acid used by the body to produce the neurotransmitters norepinephrine and dopamine, which promote alertness. It can alleviate depression, improve memory and mental alertness, increase sexual interest, and reduce hunger.

Phenytoin (Dilantin). Antiseizure medication that is useful in low doses to improve concentration, mood, and general cognitive function.

Phosphatidylcholine. A type of phospholipid (fat) that plays a major role in determining the integrity and fluidity of brain-cell membranes. It also helps relay chemical messages between neurons, and stimulates the production of the neurotransmitters dopamine, norepinephrine, and serotonin.

Phosphatidylserine. A type of phospholipid that plays a major role in determining the integrity of brain-cell membranes. It also helps relay chemical messages between neurons, and stimulates the production of the neurotransmitters dopamine, norepinephrine, and serotonin.

Phospholipid. A type of fat that is the chief component of cell membranes and is prevalent in nerve tissue. Phosphatidylcholine and phosphatidylserine are phospholipids.

Phosphorus. A mineral that is widely distributed in the enzyme systems of the body. It is a component of bone. Phosphorus is present as phosphate in many food preservatives and carbonated beverages. An excess of it can be harmful.

Phytochemicals. Compounds occurring naturally in plant foods that have powerful protective activity in the body. Examples include lutein in leafy greens, allicin in garlic, and lycopene in tomatoes.

Pineal gland. A tiny structure in the brain that secretes melatonin. It is involved in regulating the body clock and influencing reproductive function.

Piracetam. A drug that enhances mental function by improving communication between the right and left hemispheres of the brain, increasing the brain's energy reserves, and raising acetylcholine levels.

Pituitary gland. A tiny structure in the brain that functions as a part of both the endocrine and nervous systems. It secretes at least nine major hormones that are involved in a variety of body functions.

Polyunsaturated fat. Dietary fat found in fatty fish, nut butters, and vegetable oils. It has a flexible structure and high biological activity, and is a source of essential fatty acids that are crucial for optimal brain function and the formation of cell membranes and prostaglandins.

Pons. The portion of the brain stem that provides a link between the upper and lower levels of the central nervous system.

Potassium. A mineral found primarily inside the cells. It is particularly important in glucose metabolism, kidney function, muscle (including heart muscle) action, transmission of impulses along nerves, and water and fluid balance.

Pregnenolone. A precursor hormone from which DHEA, estrogen, testosterone, and other hormones are made. It helps enhance memory, protect nerve cells, and stabilize emotions.

Progesterone. A hormone produced by the ovaries that works with estrogen to regulate the menstrual cycle. It is also produced in the central nervous system and stimulates the formation of the protective myelin sheaths that cover the nerves.

Proline. A nonessential amino acid that enhances fat metabolism and aids in the production of connective tissue.

Prostaglandins. Powerful hormonelike chemical messengers that are produced in most tissues of the body from essential fatty acids. They help regulate blood pressure, heart function, hormone synthesis, inflammation, and nerve transmission.

Proteins. Large molecules made of twenty amino acids. Eight of these, considered *essential,* cannot be synthesized in the body even though they are necessary for life, and must be consumed from sources outside the body.

Pyridoxine (vitamin B$_6$). This vitamin in the B family is necessary for the metabolism of amino acids and aids in the formation of blood cells and the synthesis of nucleic acids. It is an important factor in many cellular reactions.

Resistance reaction. This is the second phase of the stress response where the levels of cortisol rise dramatically, promoting the breakdown of proteins, the elevation of blood pressure, and the loss of magnesium, potassium, and other essential nutrients. *See* Stress response.

Reticular formation. A region of the brain stem that is responsible for helping to control motor activity, maintain arousal in the higher brain (the cerebral cortex), and relay significant sensory input to the cortex.

Riboflavin (vitamin B₂). This water-soluble vitamin in the B family is important for body growth, red cell production, and releasing energy from carbohydrates.

Right hemisphere. The right side of the cerebrum. This hemisphere controls the left side of the body and is the dominant region for emotion, facial recognition, intuition, visual/spatial skills, and the appreciation of art and music in the majority of people.

St. John's wort. An herb (*Hypericum perforatum*) that is used therapeutically to relieve depression. Studies have shown it works as well as certain prescription antidepressants, without the side effects.

Saturated fat. A type of fat found in animal products and tropical oils that has a rigid chemical structure and is solid or semisolid at room temperature. Excess saturated fat in the diet promotes obesity, and subsequently, heart disease.

Selective serotonin reuptake inhibitor (SSRI). A drug, such as Prozac, that increases levels of circulating serotonin—a neurotransmitter intimately involved in the regulation of mood and sleep. SSRIs have the potential for serious side effects, including aggression, restlessness, and suicidal thoughts.

Selegiline. The active ingredient in a drug (Deprenyl) used to treat Parkinson's disease.

Selenium. A mineral that works with glutathione peroxidase to prevent damage by free radicals. It is involved in the metabolism of eicosanoids (essential fatty acids) and it protects cell membranes from attack by free radicals. It can aid in the production of thyroid hormones, fight against environmental pollutants, and also protect lipids from oxidation (rusting), which helps prevent cardiovascular disease.

Sensory cortex. The portion of the cerebrum in which information from the five senses enters awareness.

Serotonin. A neurotransmitter that plays a key role in regulating mood and sleep. Low levels are associated with depression and insomnia.

Short-term memory. *See* Working memory.

Smart drugs. *See* Nootropics.

SSRI. *See* Selective serotonin reuptake inhibitor.

Standardized extract. An herbal supplement that has been verified to contain a certain percentage of one or more of the herb's active ingredients.

Stress response. A series of biochemical and physiological reactions initiated by the hypothalamus when the brain perceives danger or a threat. This is usually a short-lived phenomenon, but can become chronic when there are persistent stressors.

Strokes. Cerebrovascular accidents (brain attacks) in which brain function is lost due to severe disruption of blood and oxygen to the brain.

Substantia nigra. The dark-colored area located deep within the cerebrum that is rich in the hormone melatonin, the precursor to the neurotransmitter dopamine.

Synapse. The gap between two neurons (or between a neuron and an organ) across which nerve impulses are transmitted.

Tau. A protein that is the main component of the neurofibrillary tangles of Alzheimer's disease.

Taurine. An amino acid that regulates neurotransmitters. It aids in maintaining clear blood vessels and stabilizing heart rhythm.

Temporal lobe. The portion of the cerebrum that contains the centers for smell and hearing, as well as areas for memory and learning.

Testosterone. A steroid hormone that increases male characteristics.

Thalamus. The region of the brain that plays a key role in arousal, learning, memory, motor activities, and sensations, and serves as the gateway to the cerebral cortex.

Thiamine (vitamin B$_1$). This B vitamin is involved in the metabolism of carbohydrates to glucose. It aids in energy production, helps to alleviate symptoms of stress, and is necessary for the normal functioning of the heart, muscles, and nervous system.

Thyroid gland. This gland, located at the base of the throat, controls metabolism, the rate at which the body uses energy.

Thyroid hormones. These hormones are secreted by the thyroid gland and regulate metabolism in every cell of the body. Deficiencies result in depression, lethargy or fatigue, and impaired memory and concentration. Excess thyroid (hyperthyroid) leads to heat intolerance, nervousness, restlessness, menstrual irregularities, and weight loss.

Tocopherol (vitamin E). A potent, fat-soluble antioxidant that works synergistically with selenium. It helps maintain normal blood glucose levels, and helps prevent cancers of the gastrointestinal tract by inhibiting the conversion of nitrates to carcinogenic nitrosamines; it prevents the formation of blood clots, and reduces the susceptibility of low-density lipoproteins to oxidation (rusting).

Trans-fatty acid. A harmful substance produced when vegetable oil is heated and chemically treated to make it solid at room temperature. These fats are linked to cancer, diabetes, heart disease, and high cholesterol.

Transient ischemic attack (TIA). A brief episode of cerebrovascular insufficiency caused by partial blockage of an artery to the brain; also called a ministroke.

Tryptophan. An amino acid that is converted in a two-step process into the neurotransmitter serotonin. Used for its antidepressant and sleep-promoting qualities, tryptophan is currently available through compounding pharmacies by prescription only.

Tyrosine. An amino acid that is involved with neurotransmitters. It helps to alleviate depression and stress.

Unsaturated fat. The type of fat found in vegetable oils that has a flexible chemical structure and is liquid at room temperature. *See also* Monounsaturated fat, Polyunsaturated fat.

Valerian. An herb that promotes sleep without causing daytime sleepiness or an impairment in mental or physical performance.

Vinpocetine. A plant-derived nootropic that improves blood flow and oxygen supply to the brain, and protects neurons from the harmful effects of hypoxia. It is used as a therapy for cerebral vascular insufficiency, as well as epilepsy and symptoms of senile dementia.

Wernicke's area. The portion of the brain involved in speech comprehension.

Working memory. Also called short-term memory, the working memory temporarily holds bits of information from a few seconds to a few hours.

Xenobiotic. A chemical or substance that is foreign to an organism or biological system.

Zinc. An essential trace mineral and a component of more than two hundred enzymes. It can increase the level of T cells in individuals over seventy, and it is involved in cellular division, growth, and repair. It helps prevent prostate gland dysfunction in older men, helps prevent vision loss due to macular degeneration and cataracts, and stabilizes cell membranes against free-radical damage, thereby boosting immunity.

Resources

Administration on Aging
Department of Health and Human
  Services (DHHS)
330 Independence Avenue SW
Washington, DC 20201
Ph: 202-619-7501 or 800-677-1116
Fax: 202-619-0724
Website: www.aoa.dhhs.gov
e-mail: aoainfo@aoa.gov

Alliance for Aging Research
2021 K Street NW, Suite 305
Washington, DC 20006
Ph: 202-293-2856
Fax: 202-785-8574
Website: www.agingresearch.org
e-mail: info@agingresearch.org

**American Association of Retired
  Persons**
601 E Street NW
Washington, DC 20049
Ph: 202-434-227 or 800-424-3410
Fax: 202-434-7599
Website: www.aarp.org
e-mail: members@aarp.org

American Geriatrics Society
350 Fifth Avenue
New York, NY 10118

Ph: 212-308-1414
Fax: 212-832-8646
Website: www.americangeriatrics.org
e-mail:
  info.amger@americangeriatrics.org

American Society on Aging
833 Market Street, Suite 511
San Francisco, CA 94103
Ph: 415-974-9600 or 800-537-9728
Fax: 415-974-0300
Website: www.asaging.org
e-mail: info@asaging.org

**Gerontological Society of
  America**
1030 Fifteenth Street NW,
  Suite 250
Washington, DC 20005
Ph: 202-842-1275
Fax: 202-842-1150
Website: www.geron.org
e-mail: geron@geron.org

National Council on the Aging, Inc.
409 Third Street SW, Suite 200
Washington, DC 20024
Ph: 800-896-3650
Fax: 301-942-2302
Website: www.ncoa.org
e-mail: info@thefamilycaregiver.org

ALZHEIMER'S DISEASE

Alzheimer's Association
919 North Michigan Avenue,
  Suite 1100
Chicago, IL 60611
Ph: 312-335-8700 or 800-272-3900
Fax: 866-699-1246
Website: www.alz.org
e-mail: info@alz.org

**Alzheimer's Disease Education
and Referral Center**
P.O. Box 825
Silver Spring, MD 20907
Ph: 800-443-2273 (English and
  Spanish)
Fax: 410-546-0184
Website: www.alzheimers.org
e-mail: adear@alzheimers.org

**American Health Assistance
Foundation**
15825 Shady Grove Road, Suite 140
Rockville, MD 20850
Ph: 301-948-3244 or 800-437-2423
Fax: 301-258-9454
Website: www.ahaf.org
e-mail: info@ahaf.org

GENERAL HEALTH

**American Academy of Family
Physicians**
1400 Tomahawk Creek Parkway
Leawood, KS 66211
Ph: 913-906-6000 or 800-274-2237
Fax: 913-906-6094
Website: www/aafp.org
e-mail: fp@aafp.org

American College of Physicians
American Society of Internal Medicine
190 North Independence Mall West
Philadelphia, PA 19106
Ph 215-351-2801 or 800-523-2400
Fax: 215-351-2829
Website: www.acponline.org
e-mail: interpub@mail.acponline.org

American Medical Association
515 North State Street
Chicago, IL 60610
Ph: 312-4650 or 800-621-8335
Fax: 800-262-3211
Website: www.ama-assn.org
e-mail: msc@ama.assn.org

**American Pharmaceutical
Association**
2215 Constitution Avenue NW
Washington, DC 20037
Ph: 202-628-4410 or 800-237-2742
Fax: 202-783-2351
Website: www.pharmacyandyou.org
  (consumer information site)
e-mail: webmaster@mail.aphanet.org

**National Council on Patient
Information and Education**
4915 Saint Elmo Avenue, Suite 505
Bethesda, MD 20814
Ph: 301-656-8565
Fax: 301-656-4464
Website: www.talkaboutrx.org

National Library of Medicine
National Institutes of Health
Bethesda, MD 20894
Ph: 301-496-6308 or 888-346-3656
Fax: 301-402-1384
Website: www.nlm.nih.gov
e-mail: custserv@nlm.nih.gov

HEALTHY LIFESTYLE

Center for the Study of Aging/ International Association of Physical Activity, Aging, and Sports
705 Madison Avenue
Albany, NY 12208
Ph: 518-465-6927
Fax: 518-462-1339
Website:
www.centerforthestudyofaging.org
e-mail:
csa@centerforthestudyofaging.org

National Association for Health and Fitness
65 Niagara Falls Square
Room 607
Buffalo, NY 14202
Ph: 716-583-0521
Fax: 716-851-4309
Website: www.physicalfitness.org

National Senior Games Association
3032 Old Forge Drive
Baton Rouge, LA 70808
Ph: 225-925-5678
Fax: 225-766-9115
Website: www.nsga.com
e-mail: nsqa@nsqa.com

HEARING

American Speech-Language-Hearing Association
10801 Rockville Pike
Rockville, MD 20852
Ph: 800-498-2071 or 800-638-8255;
TTY: 800-638-8255
Fax: 240-333-4705
Website: www.asha.org
e-mail: actioncenter@asha.org

MENTAL HEALTH

American Association for Geriatric Psychiatry
7919 Woodmont Avenue,
Suite 1050
Bethesda, MD 20814
Ph: 301-654-7850
Fax: 301-654-4137
Website: www.aagpgpa.org
e-mail: main@aagponline.org

American Psychiatric Association
1400 K Street NW
Washington, DC 20005
Ph: 703-907-7300
Fax: 703-907-1085
Website: www.psych.org
e-mail: apa@psych.org

American Psychological Association
750 First Street NE
Washington, DC 20002
Ph: 202-336-5500 or 800-374-2721
Fax: 202-336-5502
Website: www.apa.org
e-mail: webmaster@apa.org

National Institute of Mental Health
National Institutes of Health
Bethesda, MD 20892
Ph: 800-412-4211
Fax: 301-718-6366
Website: www.nimh.nih.gov
e-mail: nimhinfo@nih.gov

NEUROLOGICAL

American Academy of Neurology
1080 Montreal Avenue
St. Paul, MN 55116
Ph: 651-695-1940
Fax: 651-695-2791
Websites: www.aan.com and
   www.neurology.org
e-mail: memberservices@aan.com

**The Dana Alliance for Brain
   Initiatives**
745 Fifth Avenue, Suite 700
New York, NY 10151
Ph: 212-223-4040
Fax: 212-317-8721
Website: www.dana.org

**National Institute of Neurologial
   Disorders and Stroke**
P.O. Box 5801
Bethesda, MD 20824
Ph: 301-496-5751 or 800-352-9424
Fax: 301-402-2186
Website: www.ninds.nih.gov
e-mail: braininfo@ninds.nih.gov

National Stroke Association
9707 East Easter Lane
Englewood, CO 80112
Ph: 303-754-0930 or 800-787-6537
   (800-STROKES)
Fax: 303-649-1328
Website: www.stroke.org

NUTRITIONAL WELL-BEING

American Dietetic Association
216 West Jackson Boulevard
Chicago, IL 60606
Ph: 312-899-0040 or 800-366-1655
   (Consumer Nutrition Hotline)

Fax: 312-899-4873
Website: www.eatright.org
e-mail: foundation@eatright.org

**Food and Nutrition Information
   Center**
Department of Agriculture
10301 Baltimore Avenue, Room 304
Beltsville, MD 20705
Ph: 301-504-5755
Website: www.nal.usda.gov
e-mail: fnic@nal.usda.gov

**National Association of Nutrition
   and Aging Service Program**
1101 Vermont Avenue NW, Suite 1001
Washington, DC 20005
Ph: 202-682-6869
Fax: 202-223-2099
Website: www.nanasp.org
e-mail: lhoward@matzblancato.com

SPECIFIC ILLNESSES

**National Institute of Arthritis
   and Musculoskeletal and
   Skin Diseases**
P.O. Box AMS
9000 Rockville Pike
Bethesda, MD 20892
Ph: 301-495-4484
Fax: 301-717-6366
Website: www.niams.nih.gov
e-mail: niamsinfo@mailnih.gov

National Cancer Institute
Office of Cancer Communications
Building 31, Room 10A16
9000 Rockville Pike
Bethesda, MD 20892
Ph: 800-422-6237 (800-4-CANCER)
Website: www.cancer.gov
e-mail: cancergovstaff@mail.nih.gov

American Diabetes Association
1701 North Beauregard Street
Alexandria, VA 22311
Ph: 703-549-1500 or 800-232-3472
    (800-DIABETES)
Fax: 703-549-6995
Website: www.diabetes.org
e-mail: membership@diabetes.org
    Or for questions:
    AskADA@diabetes.org

National Diabetes Information
    Clearinghouse
1 Information Way
Bethesda, MD 20892-3560
Ph: 301-654-3327
Fax: 301-907-8906
Website: www.niddk.nih.gov/health/
    diabetes/diabetes.htm
e-mail: ndic@info.niddk.nih.gov

National Digestive Diseases
    Information Clearinghouse
2 Information Way
Bethesda, MD 20892-3570
Ph: 301-654-3810
Fax: 301-907-8906
Website: www.niddk.nih.gov/health/
    digest/digest/htm
e-mail: nidde@info.niddk.nih.gov

American Heart Association
7272 Greenville Avenue
Dallas, TX 75231
Ph: 800-242-8721 (800-AHA-USA1)
    or 888-478-7653 (888-4-STROKE)
Website: www.americanheart.org

National Heart, Lung, and Blood
    Institute Information Center
P.O. Box 30105
Bethesda, MD 20824-0105
Ph: 301-592-8573 or 800-575-9355
Fax: 301-251-1223
Website: www.nhlbi.nih.gov/
    index.htm
e-mail: nhlbiinfo@nhlbi.nih.gov

American Parkinson's Disease
    Association
1250 Hylan Boulevard, Suite 4B
Staten Island, NY 10305
Ph: 800-223-2732
Fax: 718-981-4399
Website: www.apdaparkinson.org
e-mail: info@apdaparkinson.org

Weight-Control Information
    Network
1 Win Way
Bethesda, MD 20892-3665
Ph: 202-828-1025 or 877-946-4627

VISION CARE

American Academy of
    Ophthalmology
P.O. Box 7424
San Francisco, CA 94120
Ph: 415-561-8500 or 800-222-3937
Fax: 415-561-8567
Website: www.eyenet.org

American Optometric Association
243 North Lindbergh Boulevard
St. Louis, MO 63141
Ph: 314-991-4100 or 800-365-2219
Fax:1-314-991-4101
Website: www.aoanet.org

PRODUCTS

J. R. Carlson Laboratories, Inc.
15 College Drive
Arlington Heights, IL 60004
Ph: 800-323-4141 or 888-234-5656
Fax: 847-255-1605
Website: www.carlsonlabs.com
e-mail: carson@carlsonlabs.com
Excellent source of supplements.

American Health Foundation
1 Dana Road
Valhalla, NY 10595
Ph: 914-592-2600
Website: www.smokershistory.com

Forward Nutrition, Inc.
Customer Service Center
P.O. Box 6000
Kearney, WV 25430
Ph: 800-722-8008
Fax: 304-728-7245
Website: www.drwhitaker.com
This is a source of high-quality supplements.

Life Enhancement Products, Inc.
P.O. Box 751390
Petaluma, CA 94975
Ph: 800-543-3873
Fax: 707-769-8016
Website: www.life-enhancement.com
e-mail: info@life-enhancement.com
*This is a source of vitamins, minerals,
nootropics, and other nutrients.*

Life Extension
1100 West Commercial Boulevard
Ft. Lauderdale, FL 33309
Ph: 800-208-3444
Fax: 954-202-7743
Website: www.lef.org
This is a source for vitamins.

Vitamin Research Products
3579 Highway 50 East
Carson City, NV 89701
Ph: 800-877-2447 (800-VRP-24HR)
Website: www.vrp.com
e-mail: mail@vrp.com
*This is a source of vitamins, minerals,
nootropics, and other nutrients.*

COMPOUNDING PHARMACIES

International Academy of Compounding Pharmacies (IACP)
P.O. Box 1365
Sugarland, TX 77487
Ph: 800-927-4227
Website: www.iacprx.org

Medaus Pharmacy and Compounding Center
2637 Valleydale Road, Suite 200
Birmingham, AL 35244
Ph: 800-526-9183
Fax: 800-526-9184
Website: www.medaus.com

Professional Compounding Centers of America (PCCA)
9901 South Wilcrest
Houston, TX 77099
Ph: 800-331-2498
Fax: 800-874-5760
Website: www.pccarx.com

Women's International Pharmacy
12012 N. 111th Avenue
Youngtown, AZ 85363
Ph: 800-279-5708
Fax: 608-221-7819
Website:
www.womensinternational.com
e-mail:
info@womensinternational.com

PHYSICIAN REFERRALS

American Academy of Anti-Aging Medicine
1510 West Montana Street
Chicago, IL 60614
Ph: 773-528-4333
Fax: 773-528-5390
Website: www.worldhealth.net
e-mail: info@worldhealth.net

American College for Advancement in Medicine (ACAM)
23121 Verdugo Drive, Suite 204
Laguna Hills, CA 92653
Ph: 800-532-3688
Fax: 949-455-9679
Website: www.acam.org

References

CHAPTER 1

Baddeley, A. "The Episodic Buffer: A New Component of Working Memory?" *Trends in Cognitive Sciences.* 4(12):417–423, 2002.

Black, JE. "How a Child Builds Its Brain: Some Lessons from Animal Studies of Neural Plasticity." *American Journal of Preventive Medicine.* 27:168–171, 1998.

Carpenter, M, ed. *Coretext of Neuroanatomy,* 4th ed. Philadelphia, PA: Williams and Wilkins, 1991.

Kempermann, G. "Why New Neurons? Possible Functions for Adult Hippocampal Neurogenesis." *Journal of Neuroscience.* 22(3):635–638, 2002.

Lee, AL, et al. "Stress and Depression: Possible Links to Neuron Death in the Hippocampus." *Bipolar Disorders.* 4(2):117–128, 2002.

Mesulam, MM. *Principles of Behavioral and Cognitive Neurology.* Oxford, England: Oxford University Press, 2002.

Rolls, ET. "Memory Systems in the Brain." *Annual Review of Psychology.* 51:599–630, 2000.

Squire, LR. "Memory and the Hippocampus: A Synthesis from Findings with Rats, Monkeys and Humans." *Psychological Review.* 99:195–231, 1992.

Unlerleider, LG. "Functional Brain Imaging Studies of Cortical Mechanisms for Memory." *Science.* 270:769–775, 1995.

Victoroff, J. "The Evolution of Aging-Related Brain Change." *Neurobiology of Aging.* 20:431–435, 1999.

CHAPTER 2

Boyer, R, et al. "Asymmetric Dimethylarginine (ADMA): A novel risk factor for endothelial dysfunction: its role in hypercholesterolemia." *Circulation.* 18:1842–1847, 1998.

Brattstrom, L, et al. "Hyperhomocysteinemia in Stroke: Prevalence, Cause and Relationships to Type of Stroke and Stroke Risk Factors." *European Journal of Clinical Investigations.* 22:214–221, 1992.

Fiber, J. "Carotid Artery Stenosis—A Marker or Cause of Cognitive Dysfunction?" *Neurology Reviews.* 9(6):35–36, 2001.

Iadecola, C and Gorelick, PB. "Converging Pathogenic Mechanisms in Vascular and Neurodegenerative Dementia." *Stroke.* 34 :335–337, 2003.

Ivan, CS, Seshadri, S, et al. "Dementia after Stroke: The Framingham Study." 35:1264–1268, 2004.

Hak, EA, et al. "Perspective Study of Plasma Carotinoids and Tocopherols in Relation to Risk of Ischemic Stroke." *Journal of Stroke.* 35:1584, 2004.

Miller, AL, et al. "Homocysteine Metabolism: Nutritional Modulation and Impact on Health and Disease." *Alt. Med. Rev.* 2(4):234–254, 1997.

Plum, F and Pulsinell, W. *Cerebrovascular Disease.* New York, NY: Raven Press, 1985, 161–171.

Rundek, J, et al. "Atorvastatin Decreases Coenzyme Q_{10} Level in the Blood of Patients at Risk Cardiovascular Disease and Stroke." *Archives of Neurology.* 16: 884–892, 2004.

Weber, C, et al. "Anti-oxidative effect of dietary Coenzyme Q_{10} in Human Blood Plasma." *International Journal of Vitamin and Nutrition Research.* 64(4):311–315, 1994.

CHAPTER 3

Aisen, PS and Davis, KL. "Inflammatory mechanisms in Alzheimer's disease: implications for therapy." *American Journal of Psychiatry.* 8(151):1105–1113, 1994.

Amaducci, L. "Phosphatidylserine in the Treatment of Alzheimer's Disease: Results of a multi-center study." *Psychopharmacology Bulletin.* 24(1)134–136, 1988.

Amaducci, L, et al. "Use of Phosphatidylserine in Alzheimer's Disease." *Annals of the New York Academy of Sciences.* 640:245–249, 1991.

Bains, JS and Shaw, CA. "Neurodegenerative Disorders in Humans: The Role of Glutathione in Oxidative Stress-Mediated Neuronal Death." *Brain Research Reviews.* 25(3):335–358, 1997.

Birkmayer, JGD. "Coenzyme Nicotinamide Adenine Dinucleotide—New Therapeutic Approach for Improving Dementia of the Alzheimer Type." *Annals of Clinical and Laboratory Science.* 26(1):1–9, 1996.

Breteler, M. "Vascular Involvement in Cognitive Decline and Dementia: Epidemiologic evidence from the Rotterdam Study and the Rotterdam Scan Study." *Annals of the New York Academy of Science.* 903:457–465, 2000.

Burns, A. "Mild Cognitive Impairment in Older People." *The Lancet.* 360:1963–1965, 2002.

Cartorina, M, and Ferraris, L. "Acetyl-L-Carnitine Affects Aged Brain Receptoral System in Rodents." *Life Science.* 54(17):1205–1214, 1994.

Clark, R, Smith, AD, Jobst, DA, et al. "Folate, Vitamin B_{12}, and Serum Total Homocysteine Levels in Confirmed Alzheimer's Disease." *Archives of Neurology*. 55: 1449–1455, 1998.

Cumings, JL. "Current Perspectives in Alzheimer's Disease." *Neurology*. 51:51, 1998.

Demetriades, AK. "Functional Neuroimaging in Alzheimer's Type Dementia." *Journal of Neurological Science*. 203:247–251, 2002.

Fungfeld, EW, et al. "Double-Blind Study with Phosphatidylserine (PS) in Parkinsonian Patients with Senile Dementia of Alzheimer's Type (SDAT)." *Progress in Clinical and Biological Research*. 317:1235–1246, 1989.

Goodman, A. "Statins Are Promising Therapeutic Tools for Alzheimer's Disease." *Neurology Today*. 2(3): 22–25, 2002.

Jagust, WJ. "Neuroimaging in Dementia." *Neurologic Clinics*. 18:885–902, 2002.

Ketonen, LM. "Neuroimaging of the Aging Brain." *Neurologic Clinics*. 16:581–598, 1998.

Martin, JB. "Molecular Basis of the Neurodegenerative Disorders." *The New England Journal of Medicine*. 340(25):1970–1980, 1999.

O'Brien, J and Barber, B. "Neuroimaging in Dementia and Depression." *Advances in Psychiatric Treatment*. 6:109–119, 2000.

Pettegrew, JW, et al. "Clinical and Neuro Chemical Effects of Acetyl-L-Carnitine in Alzheimer's Disease." *Neurobiology of Aging*. 16:1–4, 1995.

Richie, K, et al. "The Dementias." *The Lancet*. 360:1759–1766, 2002.

Seshadri, S, et al. "Plasma Homocysteine as a Risk Factor for Dementia and Alzheimer's Disease." *The New England Journal of Medicine*. 346(7):476–483, 2002.

CHAPTER 4

Aarsland, Tandberg, et al. "Frequency of Dementia in Parkinson Disease." *Archives of Neurology*. 53:538–542, 1996.

Birkmayer, JGD, et al. "Nicotinamide Adenine Dinucleotide (NADA)—A New Therapeutic Approach to Parkinson's Disease: Comparison of Oral and Parenteral Application." *ACTA Neuroligica Scandinavica*. 87(46):32–35, 1993.

De Boer, AG, Sprangers, MA, et al. "Predictors of Health Care Use in Patients with Parkinson's Disease: A Longitutional Study." *Movement Disorders*. 14(5):772–779, 1999.

Haas, R. "CoQ_{10} Slows Functional Decline in Parkinson's Disease." *Archives of Neurology*. 59:1541–1550, 2002.

Shults, CW, Beal, MF, Fontaine, K, et al. "Absorption Tolerability and Effects on Mitochondrial Activity of Oral Coenzyme Q_{10} in Parkinson's Patients." *Neurology*. 50:793–795, 1998.

CHAPTER 5

Christen, Y. "Oxidative Stress and Alzheimer Disease." *American Journal of Clinical Nutrition.* 71:621S–629S, 2000.

Cottrell, DA, et al. "Mitochondrial DNA Mutations in Disease and Aging." *Novartis Foundation Symposium.* 235:234-243, 2001.

De Benedictis, G, et al. "Inherited Variablility of the Mitochondrial Genome and Successful Aging in Humans." *Annals of the New York Academy of Science.* 908:208–218, 2000.

Green, RC. "Risk Assessment for Alzheimer's Disease with Genetic Susceptibility Testing: Has the Moment Arrived?" *Alzheimer's Quarterly.* 3:208-214, 2002.

Jama, JW, et al. "Dietary Antioxidants and Cognitive Function in a Population-Based Sample of Older Persons, The Rotterdam Study." *American Journal of Epidemiology.* 144: 275-280, 1991.

CHAPTER 6

Annadora, J, et al. "Food Restriction Reduces Brain Damage and Unproven Behavioral Outcomes Following Excitotoxic and Metabolic Insults." *Annals of Neurology.* 45:8-15, 1999.

Benton, David, et al. "The Impact of Long-Term Vitamin Supplementation on Cognitive Functioning." *Psychopharmacology.* 117:298-305, 1995.

Benton, David, et al. "Breakfast, Blood Glucose and Cognition." *Annual Journal of Clinical Nutrition.* 67:772-778, 1998.

Blaylock, R. *Excitotoxins: The Taste That Kills.* Santa Fe, NM: Health Press, 1997.

Bressler, J. *The Bressler Report.* FDA Report: An indictment of G. D. Searle and Co. Skokie, IL: April 25, 1977.

Jeijer, TD, et al. "Serum Carotenoids and Cerebral White Matter Lesions: The Rotterdam Study." *Journal of the American Geriatric Society.* 49:642-646, 2001.

Roberts, HJ. *Aspartame (NutraSweet), Is It Safe?* West Palm Beach, FL: Sunshine Sentinel Press, 1992.

Schmidt, MA. *Smart Fats.* Edmonton, Alberta, Canada: Frog, Ltd, 1997.

Sears, B. *Enter the Zone.* New York, NY: HarperCollins, 1995.

Stewart, HL. *Sugar Busters!* New York, NY: Ballantine Publishing Group, 1998.

CHAPTER 7

Alpert, JE, et al. "Nutrition and Depression: The Role of Folate." *Nutrition Review.* 55(5): 145-149, 1997.

Benton, D, et al. "The Impact of Long-Term Vitamin Supplementation on Cognitive Functioning." *Psychopharmacology.* 117(3):298–305, 1995.

Bertelli, A, et al. "Carnitine and Coenzyme Q_{10}: Biochemical Properties and Functions, Synergism and Complementary Action." *International Journal of Tissue Reactions.* 12(3):183–186, 1990.

Blaylock, RL. "Neurogeneration and Aging of the Central Nervous System: Prevention and Treatment by Phyto-Chemicals and Metabolic Nutrients." *Integrative Medicine.* 1(3):117–133, 1998.

Brown, R. and Colman, C. *Stop Depression Now.* New York, NY: The Berkley Publishing Group, 1999.

Clarke, R, et al. "Folate, Vitamin B_{12}, and Serum Total Homocysteine Levels in Confirmed Alzheimer Disease." *Archives of Neurology.* 55(11):1449–1455, 1998.

Crook, TH, Tinklenberg, J, and Yesavage, J. "Effects of Phosphatidylserine in Age-Associated Memory Impairment." *Neurology.* 41:644–649, 1991.

Solomon, PR, et al. "Ginkgo for Memory Enhancement: A Randomized Controlled Trial." *The Journal of the American Medical Association (JAMA).* 288(7): 835–840, 2002.

Wang, HX, et al. "Vitamin B_{12} and Folate in Relation to the Development of Alzheimer's Disease." *Neurology.* 56(9):1188–1194, 2001.

CHAPTER 8

Carson, R. *Silent Spring.* Boston, MA: Houghton Mifflin, 1962.

Eggleston, DW and Nylander, M. "Correlation of Dental Amalgam with Mercury in Brain Tissue." *Journal of Prosthetic Dentistry.* 58:704–707, 1987.

Gorell, JM, Johnson, CC, Rybicki, BA, et al. "Occupational Exposures to Metals as Risk Factors for Parkinson's Disease." *Neurology.* 48:650–658, 1997.

Le Couteur, DG, McLean, AJ, et al. "Pesticides and Parkinson's Disease." *Biomedical Pharmacotherapy.* 53:122–130, 1999.

Lorscheider, FL and Vimy, MJ. "Mercury Exposure from Silver Tooth Fillings: Emerging Evidence Questions a Traditional Dental Paradigm." *Journal of the Federation of American Societies for Experimental Biology.* 9:504–508, 1995.

——. "Serial Measurements of Intra-Oral Air Mercury: Estimation of Daily Dose from Dental Amalgam." *Journal of Dental Research.* 64:1072–1075, 1985.

Morton, WE. "Solvent Toxicity and Cognition Impairment." *Archives of Neurology.* 57:282, 2000.

Yokel, RA. "The Toxicology of Aluminum in the Brain: A Review." *Neurotoxicology.* 21:813–828, 2000.

CHAPTER 9

Buffington, CK. "DHEA: Elixir of Youth or Mirror of Age?" *Journal of the American Geriatrics Society.* 46:391–192, 1998.

Cherrier, MM, et al. "Testosterone Supplementation Improves Spatial and Verbal Memory in Healthy Older Men." *Neurology.* 57(1):80–88, 2001.

Dugbartey, AT. "Neurocognitive Aspects of Hypothyroidism." *Archives of Internal Medicine.* 158:1413–1418, 1998.

Grodstein, F, Chen, J, et al. "Postmenopausal Hormone Therapy and Cognitive Function in Healthy Older Women." *Journal of the American Geriatrics Society.* 48: 746–752, 2000.

Huether, G. "Melatonin as an Anti-Aging Drug: Between Facts and Fantasy." *Gerontology.* 42:87–96, 1996.

Hurn, PD and Macrae, IM. "Estrogen as a Neuroprotectant in Stroke." *Journal of Cerebral Blood Flow and Metabolism.* 20:631–652, 2000.

Majewska, M, et al. "Neruonal Action of DHEA: Possible Role in Brain Development, Aging, and Memory." *Annals of the New York Academy of Science.* 774:11–12, 1994.

Nelson, HD. "Postmenopausal Estrogen for Treatment of Hot Flashes: Clinical Applications." *Journal of the American Medical Association (JAMA).* 291:1621–1625, 2004.

Rako, S. *The Hormone of Desire: The Truth about Testosterone, Sexuality and Menopause.* New York, NY: Three Rivers Press, 1997.

Regelson, W. "Dehydroepiandrosterone (DHEA) the Multi-functional Steroid: Effects on the Central Nervous System, Cell Proliferation, Metabolic and Vascular Clinical and Other Effects." *Annals of the New York Academy of Science.* 564:564–575, 1994.

Regelson, W and Coleman, C. *The Superhormone Promise.* New York, NY: Simon and Schuster, 1996.

Rudman, Daniel. "Effects of Human Growth Hormone in Men over 60 Years Old." *The New England Journal of Medicine.* 323:1–6, 1990.

Shumacher, SA, et al. "Women's Health Initiative Study." *The Journal of the American Medical Association (JAMA)* 289:2651–2662, 2003.

Smoller, SW, et al. "Women's Health Initiative Study." *The Journal of the American Medical Association (JAMA).* 289:2673–2684, 2003.

Vance, ML. "Can Growth Hormone Prevent Aging?" *The New England Journal of Medicine.* 348:779–780, 2003.

Vleit, EL. *The Savvy Women's Guide to Estrogen.* Tucson, AZ: Her Place Press, 2005.

Weissel, M. "Administration of Thyroid Hormones in Therapy of Psychiatric Illnesses." *ACTA Medica Austriaca.* 26(4):129–131, 1999.

CHAPTER 10

Blake, LM. "Aging, Stress, and Affective Disorders." *Seminars in Clinical Neuropsychiatry.* 6:27–31, 2001.

Cotman, CW, et al. "Exercise: A Behavioral Intervention to Enhance Brain Health and Plasticity." *Trends in Neurosciences.* 25(6):295–301, 2002.

O'Brien, J. "Mercury Amalgam Toxicity." Interview with JK Davis. *Life Extension,* May 2001.

Myers, J, et al. "Exercise Capacity and Mortality among Men Referred for Exercise Testing." *The New England Journal of Medicine.* 346(11):793–801, 2002.

Patel, C. "Stress Management and Hypertension." *ACTA Physiologica Scandinavica Supplement L.* 640:155–157, 1997.

Sapolsky, RM. "Why Stress Is Bad for Your Brain." *Science.* 273:749–750, 1996.

Vogel, G. "New Brain Cells Prompt New Theory of Depression." *Science.* 290:258–259, 2000.

Wei, M. et al. "Relationship Between Low Cardio-Respiratory Fitness and Mortality in Normal Weight, Over Weight, and Obese Men." Lifestyle Study of the Cooper Institute of Dallas, TX. *The Journal of the American Medical Association (JAMA).* 282(16):1547–1553, 1999.

Yehuda, R. "Biology of Post-Traumatic Stress Disorder." *Journal of Clinical Psychiatry.* 62:41–46, 2001.

CHAPTER 11

Baskin, DG, Figlewicz, LD, Seeley, RJ, et al. "Insulin and Leptin: Dual Adiposity Signals to the Brain for the Regulation of Food Intake and Body Weight." *Journal of Brain Research.* 848:114–123, 1999.

Calle, EE, Rodriguez, C, Walker-Thurmond, K, et al. "Overweight, Obesity, and Mortality from Cancer in a Prospectively Studied Cohort of U. W. Adults." *The New England Journal of Medicine.* 348:1625–1638, 2003.

Dufty, W. *Sugar Blues.* New York, NY: Warner Books, 1975.

Halsted, CH. "Obesity: Effects on the Liver and Gastrointestinal System." *Current Opinions in Clinical Nutrition and Metabolic Care.* 2:425–429, 1999.

Hauri, P, Horber, FF, and Sendi, P. "Is Bariatric Surgery Worth Its Costs?" *Obesity Surgery.* 9:480–483, 1999.

Kant, AK, Schatzkin, A, Graubard, BI, et al. "A Prospective Study of Diet Quality and Mortality in Women." *The Journal of the American Medical Association (JAMA).* 283:2109–2115, 2000.

Kushner, R. "Managing the Obese Patient after Bariatric Surgery: A Case Report of Severe Malnutrition and Review of the Literature." *Journal of Parenteral and Enteral Nutrition (JPEN)*. 24:126–132, 2000.

Lappé, FM. *Diet for a Small Planet*. New York, NY: Ballantine Books, 1971.

National Task Force on the Prevention and Treatment of Obesity. *Overweight, Obesity, and Health Risk. Archives of Internal Medicine*. 160:898–904, 2000.

Ornish, D, Sherwitz, LW, Billing, JH, et al. "Intensive Lifestyle Changes for Reversal of Coronary Heart Disease." *The Journal of the American Medical Association (JAMA)*. 280:2001–2007, 1998.

Rosenbaum, RL and Leibel, JH. "Medical Progress: Obesity." *The New England Journal of Medicine*. 337:396–407, 1997.

CHAPTER 12

Aigner, C. "Advice in Health Food Stores." *Nutrition Forum*. 5:1–4, 1988.

Bartke, A, Coschigano, K, et al. "Genes that Prolong Life: Relationships of Growth Hormone and Growth to Aging and Life Span." *Journal of Gerontology, Series A: Biological Sciences and Medical Sciences*. 56:340–349, 2001.

Lovestone, S. "Diabetes and Dementia: Is the Brain Another Site of End-Organ Damage?" *Neurology*. 53:1907, 1999.

Marquis, S, et al. "Independent Predictors of Cognitive Decline in Healthy Elderly Persons." *Archives of Neurology*. 59(4):601–606, 2002.

Regelson, W and Coleman, C. *The Superhormone Promise*. New York, NY: Simon and Schuster, 1996.

Stoffer, SS, et al. "Advice from Some Health Food Stores." *The Journal of the American Medical Association (JAMA)*. 244:2045–2046, 1980.

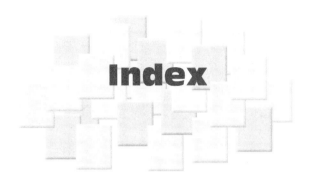

Index

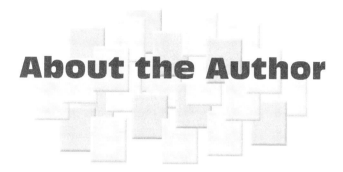

About the Author

Jordan K. Davis, M.D., a Diplomate of the American Board of Neurological Surgery, received his medical degree at the Medical College of Alabama in Birmingham, Alabama. He is the founder of the Brain and Memory Institute of America, the American Anti-Aging Foundation, the Spine Care Institute, and the Florida Back Institute. In his more than thirty years of experience observing and treating brain disorders, he has been affiliated with numerous organizations, published articles in clinical journals, and lectured at many seminars and symposia related to his field.

Dr. Davis and his wife live in Boca Raton, Florida, and Santa Fe, New Mexico. They have three grown children.